STROKES AND HEAD INJURIES:
A Guide for Patients, Families, Friends and Carers

This book offers optimism and hope to people with brain damage and the people who look after them. The authors describe the patient's possible handicaps in order to show how they can be overcome. They explain what strokes and head injuries are, who the victims may be and why, what the patient feels and can expect to feel in the future, how carers can help, and how patients can help themselves. The recovery stages are described, with practical advice on how everyone involved can help make the best of each situation.

The book is for lay people, and is written in clear language. The underlying concepts are based on the most up-to-date expertise available in the rehabilitation of brain-damaged patients. *Strokes and Head Injuries* will certainly also interest students and professionals working in this field, including physiotherapists, occupational therapists, social workers, nurses and doctors.

Mary Lynch, chartered physiotherapist, is an acknowledged expert on modern rehabilitation concepts for stroke and head injured patients. She has specialized in the treatment of neurologically damaged patients for many years. She was physiotherapist in charge of one of the largest rehabilitation units in Britain, at the Walton Hospital in Liverpool. She subsequently worked at the world-famous Bobath Centre in London, and became a qualified Bobath Tutor. As Senior Bobath Tutor, she currently organizes all the training courses run from the Bobath Centre for physiotherapists, occupational therapists and nurses, and has responsibility for teacher training in Britain and abroad. She established the pioneer courses teaching the Bobath concept in Australia, Canada, Hong Kong, Norway, Spain and Portugal. Mary Lynch lectures worldwide, travelling regularly to America, Switzerland and Germany. In 1986 and 1987 she lectured to the medical conference on the rehabilitation of stroke patients organized by the Royal College of Physicians. She holds an honorary lectureship to the Seminar College, Chester. She was founder-chairman of the Association of Chartered Physiotherapists Interested in Neurology (ACPIN), is a member of the British Stroke Research Group, and an executive of the International Bobath Instructors' Association (IBITAH). Besides her teaching commitments, Mary Lynch has a private practice in London.

Vivian Grisogono, chartered physiotherapist and health writer, has a special interest in patients with brain damage. Her first experience of their rehabilitation was gained at the Rivermead Rehabilitation Centre in Oxford. She is currently in private practice in London.

Strokes and Head Injuries

A GUIDE FOR PATIENTS, FAMILIES, FRIENDS AND CARERS

Mary Lynch
and
Vivian Grisogono

JOHN MURRAY

© Mary Lynch and Vivian Grisogono 1991

First published 1991
by John Murray (Publishers) Ltd
50 Albemarle Street, London W1X 4BD

Typeset and printed by
Butler & Tanner Ltd, Frome

British Library Cataloguing in Publication Data
Lynch, Mary
  Strokes and head injuries : a guide for patients,
  families, friends and carers.
  1. Brain damaged persons. Rehabilitation
  I. Title   II. Grisogono, Vivian
  362.1968

ISBN 0–7195–4697–4

For Robert and Andrew

Contents

Contents

Explanatory note

For clarity, we have referred to the patient (victim of a stroke or head injury) as 'him' and the therapist and carer as 'her' throughout this book, although in real life the patient may equally well be female and the therapist or carer male.

In the diagrams, the side of the patient's body affected or damaged by the stroke or head injury is represented as a shaded area.

Acknowledgements

Our very deep gratitude goes to Mrs Berta Bobath, MBE, FCSP, PhD (Hon) Boston, and to her husband Dr Karel Bobath, MD, DPM, FRCPsych. They pioneered revolutionary advances in the treatment of stroke- and head-injured patients, and have shared their knowledge and experience with countless physiotherapists who will continue their work for generations to come.

For their help with different aspects of the book we thank Margaret Baldwin, Community Stroke Nurse; Anne-Marie Boyle, Bobath Instructor; Sue Edwards, Superintendent Physiotherapist to the National Hospital of Nervous Diseases; Gerlinde Haase, Bobath Instructor; Anna Hamer, District Physiotherapist (Neurology) to the East Surrey Health Authority; Roger Hudson, editor; Michael Bartlett, artist; Dawn Bartlett and Paula Lynch.

Our special thanks are owed to the patients and their families who have kindly allowed their stories to be told in this book.

Mary Lynch
Vivian Grisogono

Chartered physiotherapists

1
What This Book Is About

Anyone who has survived a stroke or head injury is likely to have a measure of disability, sometimes mild, sometimes severe. The main physical effect of a stroke or head injury is *hemiplegia*, or damage to one side of the body. Hemiplegia causes *spasticity*, which distorts the affected side and interferes with normal movements. The physical disability may be complicated by emotional problems and difficulties with memory, understanding, speech, reading and writing. Only the lucky few recover immediately from a stroke or head injury without suffering any after-effects.

There is no operation or medicine that can cure the disabilities resulting from a stroke or head injury. Nor is it a question of time. If one simply waits for 'Time the Great Healer' to cure the patient, the disabilities get worse, and the patient becomes totally dependent on those around him for every aspect of his daily life, including washing, dressing, eating, going to the toilet and generally getting around. Therefore, it is in the best interests not only of the patient, but also of those around him, if he can be helped to recover as much as possible.

The only way the patient can overcome his disabilities is through appropriate rehabilitation. This involves expert guidance and skilled handling from professional rehabilitation practitioners and, equally important, concentrated and consistent co-operation from the patient, helped and supported by family and friends. The rehabilitation professionals involved include chartered physiotherapists, occupational therapists, speech therapists and psychologists, supported by the general practitioner and social services workers. The total care of the patient is done through co-ordination between all the professionals. There is often

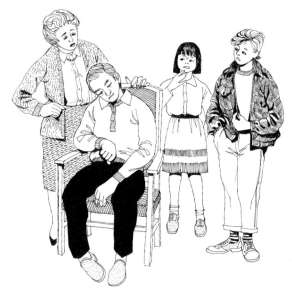

Support from family and friends is vital for the stroke or head-injured patient.

overlap in the aspects of care dealt with by each group of professionals, so to guarantee a unified approach there must be good communications between them.

The physiotherapist is usually in charge of the patient's physical rehabilitation. The rehabilitation techniques used to teach stroke and head-injured patients how to sit, move, walk and cope with daily activities safely have changed considerably over the last thirty years.

The traditional method was to do strengthening and stretching exercises for the affected arm and leg, and to allow the patient to use his unaffected side to walk and move about. Because balance was not specifically retrained in this method, the patient would almost certainly have to use a stick for support, usually a special one with three or four feet for stability (tripod or quadrupod). He would walk slowly, virtually dragging his affected leg along. It used to be customary for the physiotherapist to teach the patient how to walk, while the occupational therapist would teach him practical activities such as washing and dressing. Sometimes the physiotherapist would do exercises only for the leg, while the occcupational therapist would be in sole charge of the patient's arm exercises. If the patient had no active recovery in his affected arm, the arm might be put into a sling, even

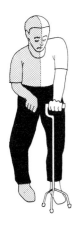

Over-compensation by the normal side leaves the patient with no real control of his movements.

though this might leave it very stiff and often painful.

This type of approach to rehabilitating stroke and head-injured patients is often referred to as the *compensatory method*. It is now considered totally outdated, because modern research has proved that the basic problem for the hemiplegic patient is the resulting spasticity, not muscle weakness, so strengthening exercises are inappropriate, because they inevitably make the spasticity worse.

Conductive education is a treatment method which was pioneered in Hungary. It was devised by Professor Andreas Peto, and practised consistently at his institute in Budapest. There is now a four-year course in the system in Hungary, leading to the qualification of 'conductor', but many qualified rehabilitation practitioners, such as physiotherapists and occupational therapists, have learned the principles and adopted them within their own methods of practice. Conductive education involves analysing functional tasks, such as the series of movements needed to drink from a cup, in order to teach the patient how to perform these movements. Teaching is done mainly in group sessions, and the patient's gradually acquired skills are reinforced by consistent practice. The patient is set reasonable targets to achieve, so he can see his own progress as he learns to do simple daily tasks. He is taught to say out loud what movement he is about to do, and then he counts aloud as he performs the movement, so that each action is given its own rhythm. This method of learning is termed *rhythmic intention*. The method was made known by the Budapest institute's world-famous successes in treating children with cerebral palsy, but in recent years it has also been applied to the treatment of adults with disabilities from brain damage.

The *motor learning programme* is another approach to treating stroke patients. Like conductive education, it is based on the principle of teaching the patient specific tasks, which he learns to perform by mastering the different movements needed for a given task bit by bit. The therapist analyses the components of a specific task, explains each action to the patient, and then asks him to do it. All the actions taught are directly related to a functional task, such as reaching forward to touch or pick up an object with the affected hand, or standing up from a chair in order to walk. The method of teaching the patient is different from the training methods used in conductive education, although the principle is similar.

The motor learning system was developed in Australia in the late 1970s, and was based on the increasing scientific evidence about what normal body movements (biomechanics) consist of, and what happens, not only physiologically but psychologically, when the body's normal actions are disrupted by the effects of a stroke. Only patients with a very good initial level of spontaneous recovery can be treated according to this method, because they need to be fully aware of what they are doing, and they need to be able to balance successfully while sitting or standing in order to achieve the functional tasks required of them. Some physiotherapists use the system as their exclusive treatment method for stroke patients, while many others incorporate some of the principles within a wider range of techniques.

The *Johnstone concept of rehabilitation after stroke* is a treatment method developed in the 1970s by British physiotherapist Margaret Johnstone. She maintains that the stroke patient needs to regain postural control by inhibiting the abnormal patterns of movement associated with spasticity. The patient has to be correctly positioned all the time to prevent spastic reactions. When the patient is properly positioned, he can do exercise routines to improve his overall physical function. To help hold the patient's hemiplegic arm and leg against the spastic forces, pressure splints, similar to the inflatable supports used by casualty workers for broken bones, hold the limbs in the required position. The original thinking underlying this treatment method has been developed through personal clinical practice. The details of the method have been publicized through several books, and are widely taught to therapists through short seminars.

The *Bobath method* was devised in the late 1940s by Mrs Berta Bobath, MBE, FCSP. With support from the Spastics Society, Mrs Bobath founded the Bobath Centre in London as a specialist charitable unit for the treatment of children with cerebral palsy. As an extension of her work with brain-damaged children, she applied her treatment methods to adult hemiplegic patients. Her treatment techniques have evolved with clinical practice, although the basic principles have not changed, and Mrs Bobath renamed her system the *Bobath concept,* to indicate that the system should not be considered fixed and stereotyped, as it could continue to develop in accordance with the modern scientific knowledge about the brain and the central nervous system. The basis of the system is that the patient can relearn normal movement by learning to control the problems resulting from a stroke or head injury, in particular the problem of spasticity. The relearning of normal postural reactions, which we take for granted, is the foundation for safe, effective movement. The therapist helps the patient by guiding him through actions and patterns of movement designed to reduce his spastic reactions, so that he can learn to use his affected arm and leg confidently for normal activities like balancing, walking, dressing and eating. The treatment system as applied to brain-damaged children is taught at the Bobath Centre in courses for doctors, physiotherapists, occupational therapists and speech therapists. The adult hemiplegia treatment system is taught world-wide in post-registration courses for qualified physiotherapists and occupational therapists. In selected countries, short courses are run for doctors, nurses and speech therapists.

This book describes the various stages of recovery and rehabilitation when someone has had a stroke or head injury. The rehabilitation principles described are largely based on the Bobath concept, and learned in practice over many years of specialization in the treatment of stroke and head-injured patients. Rehabilitation is not guaranteed to return the patient fully to normal, but it does ensure improvement and a good chance of at least some level of independent life. It involves specialist treatment: British physiotherapists with particular training in the field are usually members of the Association of Chartered Physiotherapists Interested in Neurology (ACPIN). However, rehabilitation of the stroke or head-injured patient is a twenty-four hour process, and this is why it is so important for the patient's carers, whether close family or friends, to be involved in the recovery procedures, and to learn what is right and wrong in helping him. With good rehabilitation guidance, and total co-operation between the professional workers and the carers, the patient has hope. Without this back-up, the patient is likely to sink into a wheelchair-bound torpor without hope of escape.

The detailed descriptions in this book are designed to make it easier for carers to handle the patient well and with understanding. All carers have a special role in stimulating the patient to want to get better, and in providing the right set-up for this to happen. Proper handling also, incidentally, reduces the mental and physical strain on the carer: she is much less likely to expend useless emotional or physical effort, or to injure her back, if she has learned how to give the patient effective support using modern handling techniques. Always remember, however, to consult the practitioners actually treating the patient before trying to do any handling or care on your own. If their advice seems to conflict with that given in this book, you must be guided by the practitioners, as they have the individual knowledge of the patient's case needed to give accurate care.

2
Brain Damage, Hemiplegia and Spasticity

A stroke is a sudden incident in which there is damage to the brain because of an interruption in the flow of blood to or within it. Technically, medical people often refer to a stroke as a *cerebrovascular accident* (CVA). An older term for stroke was *apoplexy*. The common result of a stroke is a disturbance of the function on one side of the body, which is technically called *hemiplegia*. The hemiplegia happens on the opposite side of the body to the side of the brain which has been damaged, so a left cerebrovascular accident causes a right-sided hemiplegia, while a right CVA disturbs the left side of the body. In rare cases, both sides of the brain are damaged together, resulting in a *bilateral hemiplegia,* or disturbance of both sides of the body. The stroke usually happens from within, often without any obvious cause. A stroke is not a heart attack. Although both are sudden, they have very different effects. The heart attack affects only the heart itself. The stroke, by contrast, because it happens in the brain, can interfere with many different aspects of the body's functions.

A head injury, which is usually caused by an external or recognizable force, can also damage the brain and cause hemiplegia. Road traffic accidents, for instance, can cause head injury through impact, when the head hits the wind-screen, side window or roof, or is hit by an object entering the car. A direct blow can cause brain damage, for instance if the person falls and the head strikes a hard surface. This type of head injury may also involve fractures to the face and/or skull, but not necessarily. A blow can cause a build-up of blood between the brain and the skull through internal bleeding (haemorrhage), damaging the brain through compression. Brain damage in a head injury can be caused indirectly as well as directly. For instance, a blow to the chin,

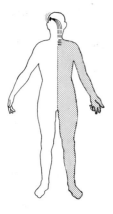

Brain damage on one side causes disruption to the other side of the body.

as in boxing, can cause reverberation of the brain within the skull, resulting in shearing damage. Similar damage can be caused by violent shaking of the head, as in the 'head-banging' craze in disco dancing.

In a stroke, the area of damage tends to be localized and clearly defined. In a head injury, the damage can be widespread, affecting many different areas of the brain. Strokes and head injuries are not the only causes of hemiplegia. Other examples are brain tumours, oxygen deprivation in the brain caused by drug overdose, and, very occasionally, multiple sclerosis, all of which can result in similar loss of balance, movement and speech.

People often mistakenly think that a stroke or head injury causes paralysis. It is true that the resulting brain damage interferes with a person's ability to move normally, but this hemiplegia should not be confused with the paralysis or total inability to move called paraplegia (both legs) or quadriplegia (trunk, both arms and both legs), both of which are caused by severe damage to the spinal cord.

In hemiplegia, whatever the cause, two main types of movement abnormality happen: *flaccidity* and *spasticity*. Both occur when the brain has lost its ability to control the spinal cord and therefore the muscles. Even when we are apparently perfectly still and relaxed, normal muscles are almost always in a state of slight tension, to counteract the effects of gravity. This constant, very low-level muscle activity is technically called *muscle tone*. Flaccidity is muscle limpness, and the patient is totally unable to activate the muscles into movement. Technically, flaccid muscles are termed *hypotonic*. Spasticity, by contrast, is over-activity in muscles which causes tightness very similar to constant cramp: the muscles seize up and resist any attempts at movement. Technically, spastic muscles are *hypertonic*. There is a third, but less common, movement abnormality called *ataxia*, which is inco-ordination of muscle activity. It is most likely to happen to patients who have had a head injury, brain tumour or drug overdose, and it makes the person look unsteady or drunk.

The stroke- or head-injured patient may suffer from either flaccidity or spasticity, or a mixture of both. The movement impairment usually affects the right or left half of the body, depending on which side of the brain the damage has occurred. The impairment may be almost imperceptible, or very severe, depending on where the damage is in the brain, and its extent. Apart from hindering normal movement, hemiplegia can also cause problems with the patient's ability to feel sensations, to speak, to understand words, to see, to eat and to control the bladder and the bowel. The head-injured patient may suffer personality changes, and adverse effects to memory and motivation. Clinical depression is a recognized problem affecting roughly 25 per cent of all hemiplegic patients. It can be due directly to the brain damage, rather than being an emotional reaction.

Normal perceptions can be altered: the patient may not be able to recognize everyday objects and their uses, and he may not realize his relationship with members of his immediate family. Our awareness of three dimensions is technically called *figure-ground* awareness: the hemiplegic patient can lose the ability to recognize whether an object is flat or round. He can be confused by spatial relationships, for instance whether things or people are above or in front of each other, so that he actually sees any group of objects as a higgledy-piggledy mass. The patient may also lose awareness of left and right, to the extent of excluding one half completely, for instance eating only half of a plateful of food, shaving only

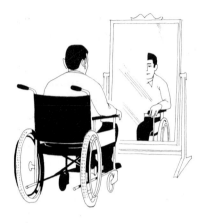

The patient may completely lose his awareness of the affected half of his body: when he looks in the mirror, he sees only the normal side.

one side of his face, or combing only half his head: this can be simply a visual problem, or it may be combined with a figure-ground problem. *Apraxia* is a special problem in which some patients lose the ability to organize their attempts at movement properly, even though they may not have lost any of their ability to move. For example, if this kind of patient were asked to get up and go into another room, he would either sit still, not knowing what to do, or he might try to comply by climbing over the back of his chair or under it in order to get up. Behaviour can appear bizarre, although it is usually totally inappropriate rather than aggressive. The majority of the most severe perceptual problems are suffered by right-handed patients who have had a right cerebrovascular accident, and therefore have a left hemiplegia. Perceptual problems are sometimes the biggest hindrance to the patient's return to normal life, and they can be the most difficult effect of hemiplegia that the carer has to understand and cope with.

The problem of spasticity

While the affected side of the patient's body may appear flaccid at first, spasticity usually sets in fairly quickly. Spasticity never changes back to flaccidity, unless the patient has another stroke or head injury. Unless it is exceptionally mild, spasticity is the biggest physical problem the patient has to overcome when recovering from hemiplegia.

The effect of spasticity is to tighten and twist the patient's hemiplegic side. The distortion causes two main recognizable patterns of body deformity: *flexor* and *extensor patterns*. In the flexor pattern, the patient's head and trunk are bent towards the affected side, with the shoulder pulled down towards the pelvis. The shoulder blade and the affected half of the pelvis are pulled backwards, making the arm and leg look shortened. The limbs are pulled in towards the body. The elbow and wrist are held bent, while the hand is clenched in a tight fist with the thumb often gripped under the fingers. The hip and knee are held bent, with the leg turned outwards. The foot is pulled up and twisted inwards. In the extensor pattern, the head pushes backwards, and the trunk is bent away from the affected side, although the shoulder girdle and flank are pulled backwards as in the flexor pattern. The affected arm is rigidly straight and turned inwards so that the palm faces backwards. The hand is either tightly fisted, or the finger tips are bent into the so-called 'monkey hand'. The leg is held forwards from the hip, with the knee straight, and is usually pulled inwards towards, or sometimes across, the other leg. The foot points downwards and inwards.

The patient has no control over the effects of spasticity on his body, which can be very complicated to understand, both for the patient and for those around him. The spasticity may be severe or mild. It can affect some parts of the body, especially the shoulder girdle, spine and hip, worse than others. There may be flaccidity in the arm or leg, for instance, combined with spasticity around the shoulder or hip. One part of the hemiplegic side may be locked into a flexor pattern, while the other may be held in the extensor pattern, or the whole side may be fixed in the same pattern. There may be pain associated with the spasticity, especially in the affected shoulder, and often in the affected wrist. The foot tends to remain painless, unless the spasticity is allowed to become established. In a tiny minority of cases, patients suffer from excruciating and unremitting pain called *thalamic pain*. This happens when the specific part of the brain called the thalamus is damaged, so that the brain no longer controls

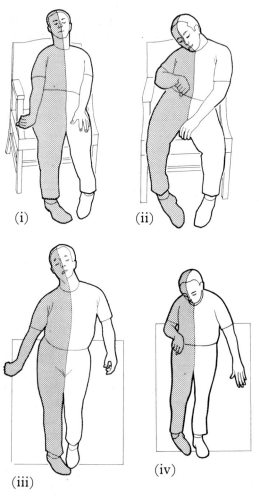

Patterns of spasticity: i Extensor pattern, sitting.
ii Flexor pattern, sitting.
iii Extensor pattern, standing.
iv Flexor pattern, standing.

the sensation messages coming to it, but interprets all sensations as pain. This means that the patient may perceive the lightest touch or different temperatures as pain sensations, so he may find it agonizing to wear clothes or even to make any kind of movement. He may be unable to be comfortable at any time. In most patients, however, the pain remains at the level of discomfort, although it is made worse by the fact that the patient cannot relieve the pain as one normally would, by stretching out or changing position.

The fixed postures produced by spasticity cannot be altered at will by the patient himself. However, he often suffers from reflex movements in the affected side, which create feelings of increased muscle tightness and body distortion. These may look like attempts at normal actions, but in fact they are entirely involuntary and abnormal, and are called *associated reactions*. They represent increasing levels of spasticity, and are triggered in a variety of different ways.

There are four major categories of associated reactions which happen without the patient's control, and usually against his will. The *extensor thrust pattern* makes the patient straighten his arms and legs hard and arch his back. If he is lying in bed, he seems to arch to lift his trunk off the bed; if he is standing up he tends to fall backwards with his body rigid. The extensor thrust reaction is triggered by stimulation or pressure to the back of the head or the trunk, for instance if the patient's head is allowed to drop back against a low pillow. The *bite reflex* is part of the extensor thrust pattern, and is especially common in head-injured patients. The patient's teeth clench together with extreme force if his head drops back. Painful sensations in his mouth can stimulate the bite reflex, for instance when his teeth are cleaned, naso gastric tubes are inserted, or waste in his mouth is suctioned out.

The second mass pattern of associated reactions is called the *positive supporting reaction*, and this is a stiffening of the leg produced in response to pressure on the ball of the foot or to stretching the sole of the foot by bending the toes upwards. The leg either straightens itself rigidly, or draws up into a tightly bent position, depending on which part of the foot has been stimulated. The third pattern is the *flexor response*, a reaction in which the hemiplegic leg automatically lifts away into a bent position. It happens when the abdominal and hip muscles are stretched, for instance if the patient tries to straighten his body as he stands up. The fourth pattern is the *grasp reflex*, in which a stimulus to the hand produces a withdrawal of the whole arm into the tightly bent (flexor) position. This happens if the patient's fingers are forcibly prised open and stretched, or if he is encouraged to grip objects such as soft spheres or rolled material in his hemiplegic hand.

Not all patients react in the same way to the same stimulus, so we cannot easily predict which mass pattern the patient might suffer. Rehabilitation treatment varies according to the individual patient's particular responses. All the handling, nursing care and treatment lines are dictated by the need to avoid stimulating the patient into uncontrollable associated reaction patterns or abnormal movements. Haphazard pressures on the patient's body are likely to trigger the most powerful reactions, which become increasingly painful and dominating, the more often they are repeated. Conversely, carefully graded repetitive stimuli of the right kind minimize the physical reflex reactions, and gradually desensitize the patient, so that these automatic responses gradually become less. This is an essential principle of the rehabilitation treatment method.

Associated reactions are a specific problem of spasticity, and they have to be carefully identified and treated. The more general problems of spasticity have to be overcome through a constant, 24-hour-a-day programme of careful handling and positioning. There are two objectives: first, to prevent the spasticity from getting worse, and second, to reduce the bad effects of the spasticity.

If the patient is left sitting or lying in a distorted position for any length of time, the spastic patterning becomes fixed, and gets worse. Lack of full support in bed, or a badly chosen chair, which leaves the hips too bent and the spine unsupported, increase the patient's spasticity. When sitting, the patient is likely to be pulled into the flexor pattern, whereas lying flat on his back his body is more likely to be fixed in the extensor pattern. When the patient is standing, his affected side might be dominated by either the flexor or the extensor pattern. Spastic postures tend to take on a life of their own, almost fighting each other for control of the hemiplegic side of the body. Once the spasticity reaches a severe and uncontrolled stage, it causes permanent deformities, called contractures.

The patient cannot fight against the stiff spastic position

to make himself comfortable without making a major effort, which in itself increases his spasticity. Emotional upsets such as tension, fear or sorrow can spark off associated reactions, making the spasticity worse. When the patient tries to roll over in bed, or pull himself up using a 'monkey bar', the combination of physical effort and frustration can increase the spasticity to the point of extreme pain, and it becomes physically impossible for him to move in any direction other than where the spastic pattern dictates. Temperature and barometric changes, or an environment which is too hot or too cold can trigger associated reactions. Automatic reflex actions such as yawning or (painful) bowel movements can also cause increased spasticity. Inappropriate handling triggers associated spastic reactions, for instance if the patient is asked to make any effort when the nurse is trying to transfer him from bed to chair, instead of being fully supported and levered up. Harsh words which upset the patient provoke increased spasticity too.

It is important to understand that the patient with spasticity cannot simply learn to use his normal side for everyday activities, and hope that the affected side will not get in the way. Any body movement automatically elicits a reaction in the spastic muscles, which, if uncontrolled, will hinder the patient's attempts to complete a given action. Spasticity can only be cured by surgery which cuts out the nerves which are sending distorted messages to the spastic muscles. While this cures the problem of unwanted abnormal reactions, it leaves the patient without any active voluntary movement at all. In some cases, this means the difference between a level of physical independence and permanent confinement to a wheelchair. In most cases, spasticity can be controlled. It is a complicated learning process, involving all the professional practitioners tending the patient, plus the family, carers and the patient himself.

Controlling spasticity is the basis of the hemiplegic patient's treatment, and the amount of control achieved determines the degree of the patient's physical recovery.

How does the brain work?

It is easier to understand why a stroke or head injury can have such varied, devastating effects when you know a little about how the brain works.

The brain is the central computer which controls all the body's functions through the nervous system. The brain and the spinal cord form the central nervous system, while the nerves which lead off from the spinal cord to the face, torso,

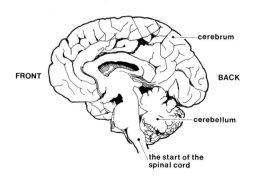

FRONT — cerebrum — BACK — cerebellum — the start of the spinal cord

Side view of the centre of the brain.

arms and legs are the peripheral nervous system.

The main upper part of the brain consists of two halves or hemispheres, known as the right and left cerebral cortex. Under the hemispheres at the back and base of the skull are two smaller parts called the right and left cerebellum. These four parts are connected to each other by the mid-brain and the brain stem. The brain stem forms the top of the spinal cord, and is therefore the bond between the central and peripheral nervous systems.

The body's functions are broadly divided into activities which can be controlled at will, such as walking, and functions which happen automatically, such as the heart beating. Different parts of the brain control different aspects of the body's activities. The cerebral cortices process the information needed when you want to perform specific movements such as kicking a ball or speaking. The cerebellum is a memory store of movement patterns which enables you to repeat accurately skills you have learned, such as writing or hitting a tennis ball with a racket. The mid-brain receives and processes the body's sensory information, such as pain, temperature, pressure and touch. The brain stem controls the automatic functions like breathing, blood flow, blood pressure and digestion.

The left side of the brain controls movement of the right side of the body, and contains the main centre for speech and understanding. The right side of the brain controls the left side of the body. It also enables you to receive and interpret information from your environment in relation to yourself. Therefore the right side of the brain is essential for judging distances, recognizing familiar people and objects, and performing everyday tasks such as dressing and washing.

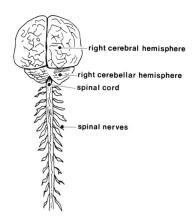

right cerebral hemisphere

right cerebellar hemisphere

spinal cord

spinal nerves

Back view of the brain and part of the spinal cord.

Each part of the brain communicates with all the other parts, plus the spinal cord. So, for the successful control of movement, your ability to feel has to be co-ordinated with your ability to move. The brain and spinal cord respond to messages from the many different parts of the body involved in movement, such as muscles, tendons, joints and skin. Proprioception is the technical name for this information. The central nervous system produces correct and appropriate movements when the information it receives is accurate. The feeling of the ground under your feet is one of the proprioceptive messages needed for you to be able to stand

17

up on two legs, even though you are not consciously aware of this sensation most of the time.

Therefore there are three parts in the mechanisms through which most body functions happen: the input to the central nervous system, the response or output which creates movement, and the feedback or relationship between the two. It is thought that flaccidity, which often occurs initially after a stroke, but may not last long before changing into spasticity, is due to spinal shock and/or swelling in the brain. Spasticity, which generally comes in as recovery starts to take place, is due to the brain's loss of control over the activity (output) of the spinal cord. Damage to the cerebellum, leading to the cerebellum's loss of control over the spinal cord, causes ataxia. It is the relationship between input and output in the central nervous system which is damaged in hemiplegia. The aim of therapy is to help the patient re-establish the link between the message systems and functional activities.

What happens in the brain when a stroke or head injury occurs?

In a stroke, the blood flow to the brain is disrupted. There are three main reasons for this. The most common is a thrombus, or blood clot, which blocks either the main carotid artery in the neck, or one of the much smaller arteries or veins in the brain. This usually happens because the artery walls have been damaged, either through trauma like a cut or a blow, or because of thickening and degeneration (technically called arteriosclerosis, atherosclerosis or atheroma, according to type). The thrombus consists of blood cells called platelets and a stringy substance called fibrinogen, which tangle together to form the clot. Sometimes the thrombus is so small that instead of blocking an artery, it passes through it, but still causes minor symptoms of a stroke. The symptoms disappear within about twenty-four hours, and leave no trace of disability or movement impairment. This is known as a transient ischaemic attack (TIA).

The second is an embolism, another type of clot (embolus) which usually lodges in the main carotid artery and therefore stops blood from reaching the brain. The embolus consists of debris from a damaged heart valve, or some other fragments, for instance an accumulation of bacteria or portions of a tumour. The debris can collect in one of the heart vessels or in the neck, and it is then rolled along by the blood stream, usually attracting more debris as it goes, so that it becomes an enlarged clot which can eventually completely plug an artery carrying blood to the brain.

The third type of blood flow interruption in a stroke is haemorrhage, or bleeding. This can happen within the substance of the brain when very tiny vessels burst or leak. This is known as a cerebral haemorrhage. Bleeding can also occur when a larger artery wall bursts. The artery wall is stretched and ballooned out by the pressure of the blood inside it, and gives way at a weak point which is either a structural defect (present from birth), or a part which has degenerated (for instance through atheroma). Technically, this is called an aneurysm.

Head injuries may cause haemorrhages or cerebral oedema (fluid swelling) within the skull and/or the brain. If the haemorrhage happens between the brain and the skull, it is called extradural, and it leads to the formation of an extradural haematoma (blood clot). Pressure from the blood clot in this confined space causes brain damage. It is often associated with a skull fracture in which the broken bone presses inwards, increasing the pressure on the brain. An intracerebral haemorrhage happens inside the brain, because of reverberation or shearing of the brain tissue. It may be widespread, causing cumulative damage.

3
Strokes and Head Injuries: Prevention and First Aid

Are strokes and head injuries preventable?

Anybody and everybody could have a stroke, because there is no absolute method of prevention. We do not (yet) have any reliable means for detecting everyone who is at risk from the various types of stroke. A stroke can happen to the very young, including babies, although strokes are most common among the over-sixties. Males and females seem to be equally vulnerable. Being born with an aneurysm in the brain does not necessarily lead to a stroke, but it gives the person the possibility of having a stroke if the aneurysm bursts. Any congenital vulnerabiity of this kind is uncontrollable.

However, there are some known factors leading to certain types of stroke which we can influence. High blood pressure is an important risk factor, so it is sensible to have your blood pressure checked by your family doctor at regular intervals if you think it might be above average. Diabetes should be well controlled, and this may entail not only taking prescribed amounts of insulin, but also regulating your diet with the help of a professional dietician. For the young diabetic who wants to do active sports, advice from the dietician is essential in establishing the correct amount and type of food needed to avoid becoming hypoglycaemic (sugar deficient).

Diet, logically, is an important aspect of our lifestyle, but there is controversy and argument over what constitutes a healthy diet, and indeed what is involved in a healthy or unhealthy lifestyle. Being overweight is likely to be 'unhealthy', especially if obesity is associated with other low-health factors, such as high blood pressure or diabetes. However, extreme or so-called 'crash' diets are unlikely to contribute to good health, partly because they rarely give lasting effects of weight loss, and partly because some of these rapid-result reducing diets deprive the body of essential nutrients needed on a daily basis. A weight-reducing diet is best undertaken under the supervision of a dietician or a recognized weight-loss clinic with a doctor in control. It is likely to be most effective when combined with a suitable exercise programme. Appropriate diet and physical exercise are now considered fundamental to our well-being.

Excessive alcohol intake has been linked to strokes. Identifying how much is too much can be a problem, if you are used to drinking wine, beer or spirits on a regular basis. Drinking alcohol to the point of becoming unconscious is an obvious sign that you have drunk to excess: anyone who drinks to this level in regular binges is likely to be at increased risk of having a stroke. However, it is also thought that even a moderate alcohol intake on a daily basis can be harmful. One possible guideline to assessing whether your alcohol intake is recognizably too high is to ask your doctor to check your liver function for signs of damage. This is done by a simple blood test.

Drugs should never be mixed with alcohol. Even mild painkillers can affect the body's systems badly in combination with liquor. Overdoses of painkillers and other therapeutic drugs can cause brain damage through oxygen starvation (anoxia): suicide attempts often result in the person surviving with severe disabilities. Hallucinatory, stimulant and narcotic drugs, when abused, can also cause brain damage. Tobacco is still a very widely used drug, even though it is known to be associated with a wide variety of diseases besides strokes. One of the best preventive measures against stroke is to give up smoking, whether cigarettes, cigars or pipe. Overcoming any addiction, especially to drugs such as cocaine and heroin, may need professional help and even treatment in special clinics, although many people manage to give up smoking habits through simpler measures such as acupuncture or using nicotine substitutes. It is, logically, an important part of health education to discourage young people, especially children, from ever taking up habits of cigarette smoking or drug abuse.

Head injuries can be prevented, to a certain extent, by taking elementary precautions in risky situations. Seat belts in cars have reduced the number of road accidents in which the head is badly injured through hitting the windscreen. Protective helmets for motorcyclists and cyclists have reduced both the numbers and the severity of head injuries when the rider comes off the bike. Road safety depends on the good sense of all road users, so pedestrians, drivers and riders alike should take special care not to put themselves and others at risk through moving about while their normal awareness is impaired, for instance through excess alcohol or painkilling drugs. If you have had even a minor injury, such as a twisted knee, you should make sure you can control your vehicle as normal before setting out on the road again. You should also remember that if you have to wear a collar for a painful neck problem, or are using crutches for a leg injury, you should not drive your car, as your temporary disability is likely to invalidate your insurance if you have an accident.

Work situations in factories and on building sites can involve head injury risks from falling objects, and it has become commonplace for workers and visitors to have to wear protective headgear. Do-it-yourself enthusiasts should use an industrial helmet if they undertake tasks such as tree lopping or ceiling and roofing work.

Many sports carry the risk of head injury, and helmets, which have been used routinely for many years in sports like American football, horse riding and men's lacrosse, are being used more widely to protect against head injury in sports such as cricket and boxing. Increased awareness of the risks is leading to a greater use of helmets for young children in sports like skiing, because the child's thin skull is specially vulnerable to damage. Protective helmets have to be properly designed and well fitting. Made-to-measure gum shields can help protect against head injury in sports like rugby or boxing, where direct blows to the chin can cause reverberations into the brain. It has to be said that as boxing is a sport which inevitably involves blows to the head which can only be partly alleviated by cushioning and protection, it is hardly surprising that many medical specialists would like to see the sport banned on the grounds that the risk of brain damage is unacceptably high. In any sport, if a player has suffered a knock to the head with even momentary

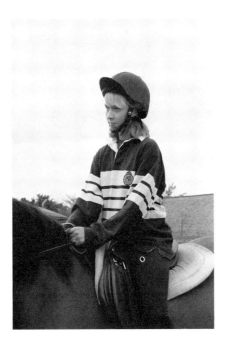

A well-fitting protective helmet is essential in sports which carry the risk of falls onto the head.

concussion, he or she should be stopped from playing on, and checked by a doctor. No player should return to sport after any head injury without being cleared by the doctor.

Physical violence always carries the risk of causing serious damage to somebody, although this is not always obvious in television and film representations of violence, when actors seem able to continue standing and moving despite flurries of heavy blows to their heads. In real life, much of this simulated television violence would result in serious head injuries and therefore death or disability for the victim. Sadly, many real-life tragedies of violence happen accidentally, for instance when a frustrated parent shakes or strikes a naughty child too harshly, causing head injury. The violent head-shaking craze in discotheque 'head-banging' is a preventable cause of possible self-inflicted head injuries, and young people should be warned against it.

As brain damage is irreversible, even though it may be possible to compensate for its effects, it has to be worth taking reasonable care to prevent strokes and head injuries.

When someone has had a stroke or head injury, it is vital to control, and if possible eliminate, the known risk factors in order to prevent further strokes or worse brain damage.

Immediate actions to take when strokes or head injuries happen

As sudden illnesses or accidents can happen anywhere, anytime, to anyone, everyone should take a standard first-aid course, in order to be able to cope in an emergency. Learning when to apply life-saving techniques, and how to do them effectively, can be the difference between life and death for a stroke or accident victim.

A minor stroke does not necessarily make the patient feel very ill, so it may not be obvious that anything much is wrong. He may or may not have a headache. He may notice his attention wandering, combined with a feeling of vagueness, as though he is 'absent' from the world around him. His speech may be slurring, and he may lose his sense of balance, wavering as he walks, or falling as he tries to get out of bed or a chair. To someone watching, he may appear drunk. He may suddenly find it difficult to formulate words, as though he had been 'struck dumb'. His eyesight may be affected, so that one side or the other of his normal field of vision may be completely blanked out. He may feel numbness or pins and needles in one hand, arm or leg, or the arm and leg on one side may be affected together. He may have difficulty moving the arm and/or leg, when he wants to perform particular actions. Even if these symptoms disappear quickly, without leaving apparent ill-effects, the sufferer should go to his family doctor for a check-up. His family or friends should encourage him to go, and preferably accompany him. If the symptoms seem to disappear immediately, the patient has probably suffered a transient ischaemic attack. If he continues to feel 'strange', and the symptoms become more pronounced, he has probably suffered a stroke. The patient should be kept comfortably at rest, and the doctor should be called to visit him as quickly as possible.

A more major stroke can happen extremely quickly or slowly, so the patient may be aware of the different sensations setting in after only a minute, or building up gradually during the space of an hour or more. Strokes often happen during sleep, so the victim may wake up and find that he cannot speak normally, has lost control over one side of his body, and perhaps has a severe headache. Although the stroke might appear to have happened out of the blue, the victim or those close to him may remember that he had noticed previous hints of the same sensations and symptoms, which had come and gone so rapidly that he had not attached any importance to them. Sometimes, raised blood pressure can cause unusual and severe nose bleeds, and this is the first warning that the victim might be at risk of having a stroke. When it is obvious that a stroke has happened, the doctor or emergency services should be called immediately. If the patient remains conscious, he should be kept calm, and encouraged to keep still and try to rest and relax. He should not be given any food or drink, in case he cannot swallow properly. He should certainly not be given any alcohol or cigarettes. If there is any delay before the arrival of the doctor or ambulance, someone should stay with the patient all the time, keeping watch in case his symptoms change or he drifts into unconsciousness.

A very major stroke usually causes unconsciousness fairly quickly, as the brain receives a shock leading to an interruption in its blood supply. If this happens when the victim is asleep, he may be found unconscious when someone tries to wake him. He may be snoring deeply, and his breathing may be laboured and irregular (technically called *Cheyne-Stoke's breathing*). His pulse may be strong but irregular and unusually slow. As the unconscious patient does not move by himself, the physical signs of the stroke, such as speech and movement difficulties, are not apparent, so it may not be obvious that brain damage has caused the victim's condition. If you gently open the patient's eyes (having washed your hands first if possible), you will see that his pupils are not the same size, nor do they react by narrowing if you move a light or torch beam in front of them.

When you find someone in this condition, you should call for emergency medical care straight away. Avoid moving the patient, if at all possible. Do not shake him violently to try to wake him up. Any further movements might increase the bleeding in his brain. If the patient fell over as he became unconscious, check carefully by looking and feeling, in case he has cut himself or suffered any broken bones. If so, you will need to apply clean dressings to any wounds. You may have to support the broken bones with bandages and splints to make them more comfortable. If he really has to be moved, perhaps because he has collapsed in the street, handle him as gently as possible, preferably between several people so that carrying him is not too difficult. In all cases, place him comfortably at rest with his head and shoulders slightly raised and his face turned to one side, or lying on one side with his head, uppermost arm and leg supported, preferably on pillows (the *recovery position*). Keep him warm. If he has false teeth, it may be wise to remove them, taking care that your hands are clean. Keep a close check on whether the patient is still breathing, and take his pulse every ten minutes or so. If possible, jot down what you see and find on a piece of paper, as this may be helpful to the emergency ambulance team who come to transfer the patient to hospital.

There is no need to do resuscitation techniques (the so-called *kiss of life*) if the patient is breathing on his own, even when he is unconscious. However, a massive sudden stroke which affects a large part of the brain can stop the patient's heartbeat and breathing, causing death. If you find the patient unconscious and not breathing, you should call for the emergency medical services, and start doing life-saving techniques immediately, even if the situation seems hopeless. Artificial respiration is the first priority, so you should clear the patient's mouth of any debris, pinch his nose shut, tilt his head back, and blow into his mouth either with your lips against his, or through a special breathing tube called an airway. Let the patient 'breathe out', then repeat the input. After a few breaths, check his pulse. If it is not beating, and the patient stills looks a blue colour, you need to start cardiac (heart) massage: start by hitting the breastbone firmly with the side of your fist three times, then place both hands, one on top of the other, over the breastbone so that you can exert gentle but firm pressure onto the chest, at the rate of about one push per second for the adult – you have to work faster for children. The standard first-aid teaching is to do fifteen pushes against the breastbone alternating with two mouth-to-mouth breaths if you are working on your own, or five heart movements to one breath if someone else is doing one part of the resuscitation. You should try to keep the life-saving effort going until the ambulance team arrives, even if you do not seem to be making any progress.

A serious head injury is usually easy to recognize, as there are external signs of the damage, such as bleeding, acute pain over the affected part of the head, and perhaps an obvious fracture in the skull. Sometimes the extent of the damage is not immediately obvious: a skull fracture may not have any bleeding directly over it, but there may be bleeding from the ears, nose or mouth. A fracture at the base of the skull may not cause any visible external bleeding at all, but clear (cerebrospinal) fluid might emanate from the ears, nose or mouth. Any head injury may be accompanied by severe damage to the neck, carrying the potential risk of total paralysis. The victim may have been involved in a road traffic accident, either as a pedestrian, a rider, or in a vehicle; he may have been the victim of a mugging or a knock-out blow in a boxing bout; he may have received a bullet wound in the head, by accident or on purpose; he may have dived head-first into shallow water; or he may have fallen and hit his head against a hard surface. The correct action to take depends on the circumstances of the accident or incident. It is vital for a companion or first-aider to be able to tell the emergency services exactly what happened to the victim at the scene of the accident.

If he is conscious, the victim may feel giddy and sick. He may have a headache, and he may have no recollection of his accident, so he is confused about what is happening to him. Even if his injury does not seem severe, he should not be allowed to continue on his way alone, as he may have suffered concussion, and this may lead to after-effects in the brain. Someone should accompany him to hospital, or stay with him until the ambulance arrives. If he is bleeding, you should stem the flow with a clean dressing, taking care not to apply excessive pressure, if there is any risk that the bone underneath the wound is broken. The victim should not be given anything to drink, although you can moisten his mouth with a wet flannel. Keep a check on his condition and level of consciousness by watching him and asking him questions.

Your information will help the casualty staff assess the possible extent of the injury. At the hospital, the victim will be checked for any skull fractures or neck damage, and even if there is no bone injury he will probably be kept in for monitoring for twenty-four hours, in case brain damage is developing slowly as a result of the head injury. The victim could develop a headache and start vomiting later on, or could even collapse into unconsciousness and stop breathing, so he should not be left alone, even after an apparently mild head injury.

In severe accidents in which the victim's spine (back or neck) might be broken, it is best not to move the victim at all before the emergency services arrive, even if he is unconscious. However, if he is having difficulty breathing, it may be necessary to turn him very gently into the recovery position. If he has suffered from concussion as the direct result of a blow to the head, he is likely to feel clammy and cold to the touch, his pulse may be feeble and fast, his breathing shallow and slow. If you open his eyes gently, the pupils are equal in size. They may be narrowed, and still react to light, or, if the concussion is severe, the pupils may be dilated (wide open) and fail to change with fluctuations of light. If there is bleeding within the skull, or a broken bone pushing down onto the brain, the victim may have compression rather than concussion, and he will be restless, hot and flushed, with a strong, slow pulse, and breathing noisily. If you look at his eyes, the pupils are likely to be uneven, with one narrower than the other. If the patient is in danger of further injury, perhaps because he is lying in the road, he has to be moved, very carefully. If possible, however, he is kept completely still and calm, and covered with a blanket or overcoat for warmth. Avoid unnecessary movements involving the head or neck: if the victim is a motorcyclist, for instance, do not try to wrench off his crash helmet. Keep a check on the patient's condition and his level of consciousness by watching him closely and constantly checking his pulse and breathing. Try to perform emergency measures, such as staunching any bleeding, without disturbing the victim's position, until the ambulance team arrives.

First-aid checklist for the unconscious patient

- Assess what has happened, or what might be wrong.
- Check whether the patient is breathing.
- Check whether his pulse is beating.
- Do resuscitation and cardiac massage, if necessary.
- Stem any bleeding.
- Check for any broken bones.
- Check his eyes, if he is breathing.
- Turn the patient into the recovery position.
- Keep the patient still and warm.
- Inform the ambulance team of what has happened.

First-aid checklist for the conscious patient

- Find out exactly what happened, and what the patient feels.
- Keep the patient still, warm and calm.
- Check for obvious injuries.
- Stem any bleeding.
- Support and cover any obvious fractures.
- Observe him for any changes of condition.
- Keep talking to him.
- Do not give him food, drink or cigarettes.
- Place him in the recovery position if he loses consciousness.
- Stay with him until medical help arrives.

4
Hospital Care: Immediate and Emergency Treatment

If the head injury or stroke is severe enough, and especially if it has caused unconsciousness, the victim is admitted to hospital through the accident and emergency services. The patient is delivered to the Accident Department (also called Casualty or A & E). Relatives may be asked to sign a form giving the medical staff permission to perform the necessary emergency care procedures. In Britain, if the patient is brought into hospital without any accompanying relatives, the doctors automatically carry out any emergency treatments they consider necessary to save the patient's life.

In some cases surgery is needed: for the stroke victim, a brain haemorrhage may be drained, or an aneurysm might be sealed off with clips; in the case of a head injury, a blood clot may have to be removed from the brain, or the patient's skull may need treatment if it is broken and pressing on the brain. There may be no need for immediate action by the doctors in the case of a mild head injury or stroke. Relatives may be worried by the patient's condition and inability to move normally, but if the patient is conscious and aware, and not in obvious danger, no emergency measures will be instituted. The patient may be admitted to the hospital for diagnosis, routine care and subsequent rehabilitation. If appropriate support services and out-patient treatment can be arranged, the patient with a very mild head injury or stroke may not be admitted, but allowed home under the care of his general practitioner.

If emergency care is needed, various actions are taken immediately. Very rarely, the patient with a severe head injury or stroke has to be resuscitated, because his heart has

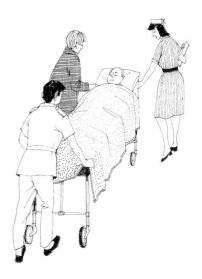

Stay close to the patient and be reassuring, even if he seems not to respond.

stopped or is beating in an abnormal rhythm. A special machine called a *defibrillator* may be used to restart the heart-beat. At the same time a tube, called an *endotracheal tube*, is inserted through the patient's mouth into the throat. The tube is attached to an oxygen cylinder, and a manually squeezed bag controls the delivery of oxygen directly to the patient's lungs. Once the heart-beat has restarted and is stabilized again, the patient may be able to breathe unaided, but he may still be kept on oxygen through a transparent face-mask, so that he can breathe more easily. If the heart is working but breathing is still difficult, the patient is attached to a *ventilator* (commonly known as a life-support machine), and usually transferred immediately to the Intensive Care (or Treatment) Unit (ICU or ITU).

For most head injury or stroke victims, resuscitation is not necessary, but other measures are needed to prevent damaging complications from developing. One of the first things that may happen is that a tube is passed through the nose into the patient's stomach. This is done if the patient is unconscious or semi-conscious, or if the stroke has impaired his ability to swallow properly. Necessary fluid and food supplements are passed directly into the stomach through the tube, which is called a *Ryle's tube* or *nasogastric tube*.

The patient may also be put on a *drip*: a needle is inserted into one of the veins in his hand, so that fluids and drugs can be passed directly into the blood stream. The needle is attached to a transparent tube which leads to a bag containing the fluid. The bag is usually suspended on a frame (drip-stand) above the patient, and a valve controls the fluid's speed of flow downwards. Drugs may be put into the bag, to be fed into the patient with the fluid, or they may be injected through a separate valve close to the needle in the hand.

The patient may have lost normal control of his bladder if he has suffered a severe head injury or stroke, or if he remains unconscious. Another tube (*catheter*) attached to a bag may be inserted into the bladder to collect the passing urine. This is done to avoid urine coming into contact with the patient's skin, as this can cause pressure sores.

Any or all of these measures might be done in the Accident Department, or later, after the patient has been admitted into hospital and transferred to one of four possible appropriate units.

If the patient is still unconscious on arrival at the hospital, the medical staff may transfer him to the Intensive Care Unit. There the patient with obvious breathing difficulties is given the right mixture of oxygen and other gases by a ventilator. This helps the brain receive the oxygen it needs for survival, and so may limit the amount of damage which would happen through further lack of oxygen. The patient is usually attached to the ventilator by a pipe (*endotracheal tube*), which is passed through the mouth, down the throat and into the windpipe (trachea) by an anaesthetist. Some-times the attachment to the ventilator goes directly into the windpipe through a surgical cut, called a *tracheostomy*. The head-injured patient is more likely to be given an immediate tracheostomy, whereas other stroke victims might be given a tracheostomy after a few days, if it seems that ventilation is likely to be needed for longer than a week or ten days.

The head-injured or stroke patient who does not need intensive emergency care, whether conscious or unconscious, may be transferred from the Accident Department to a spec-ific ward, which might be the Medical Ward, the Neuro-logical or Neurosurgical Unit, or, in a few cases, the

Orthopaedic Ward. The decision depends largely on whether the medical staff feel that the victim will need surgery or not. The patient with a very mild head injury may not seem to need hospital care, but it is normal practice for hospitals to keep these patients under observation for at least twenty-four hours in case the knock to the head causes slow-developing brain damage. On the Medical Ward the head-injured or stroke victim will be among patients with various medical problems, not necessarily strokes, and they will all be receiving medical care such as investigations and drug therapy, and nursing, perhaps including help with eating, washing and toilet needs. In the Neurological Unit the patient receives similar nursing care, but is under the neuro-surgeon who makes the decision to carry out any necessary operations. The patient with broken bones as well as a head injury might be transferred to the Orthopaedic Ward, but should normally be under the care of the neurologist as well as the orthopaedic surgeon.

In Britain the fourth option for the stroke patient's transfer is the specialist Stroke Unit. These are small hospital-based units, consisting of between ten and twenty-five beds, scattered round the country and run as part of the publicly funded National Health Service (NHS). Staffed by specially trained nurses and therapists, under medical supervision, they aim to provide a total rehabilitation programme for the stroke victim. These units are often directly involved in practical and theoretical research to identify the most common factors causing strokes, the most appropriate treatment methods and the best intensity of rehabilitation.

Admission to a Stroke Unit can be a matter of geographical luck. If the stroke victim is taken to a hospital which has a specialist unit, the patient may be referred to it directly from the Accident Department. Otherwise, referral may follow after the patient has spent a period on the Medical Ward, or after surgery on the Neurosurgical Ward. Sometimes, the stroke victim is transferred to the Stroke Unit from another hospital in the same administrative region. If relatives are informed that the victim is being transferred to another hospital, it is usually for the sake of specialist care, so it should be taken as positive news.

How relatives or companions can help in the emergency situation

When the patient is admitted to hospital, diagnostic tests are done as quickly as possible to determine why a stroke has happened, or how extensive the damage from a head injury is, and where exactly in the brain the damage from either has occurred. Some of the tests may be done in the Accident and Emergency Department, others might follow later, when the patient has been transferred to another unit. In some cases, if the hospital does not have the facilities for special tests which are considered necessary, the patient may be transferred to another, usually larger, hospital.

Relatives or friends who go to the hospital with the victim may be able to help the doctors considerably by providing background information, technically called the history. Your evidence is all the more important if the patient is unconscious, disorientated, or has lost the power of speech.

In the case of a head injury, you may be able to describe exactly what kind of accident has happened, and whether the victim has suffered even momentary loss of consciousness, memory, speech or orientation. When a stroke has occurred, there may have been warning signs during the preceding few days or weeks, such as brief black-outs, slurred speech, inattentiveness, clumsiness, stumbling or momentary loss of balance. The patient may have complained of odd sensations in one arm or leg, dizziness, vagueness or difficulty following a conversation. These symptoms may have lasted for only a few minutes, or as long as a few hours, and then appeared to vanish without leaving any ill-effects. Their description shows the doctor that the patient had probably suffered from one or more transient ischaemic attacks. There may also have been other symptoms, such as severe headaches, similar to migraine, lasting for only a couple of hours at first, but recurring later to persist for much longer. Very occasionally, before having a stroke, the patient may do things which seem completely out of character, often without any awareness or recollection of the actions.

Other useful information which the doctor may ask for concerns the patient's lifestyle, including details of drinking and smoking habits, diet, work and leisure patterns, any known worries or stresses, past and recent illnesses, medications or drugs being taken, and any known history of serious illnesses, including strokes or heart attacks, within the patient's immediate family.

In the case of stroke, the doctor also needs to know exactly how the patient's current state began. Did the victim complain of feeling unwell? If so, when? Did the attack come on suddenly or gradually? Were there any convulsions? Did the patient lose consciousness, and if so when? Did the patient breathe normally as the attack came on? Did he fall? If so, did he hit any part of the body, and which way did he fall? If the patient has suffered a known head injury, the doctor must be told exactly what happened, and whether the victim's heart or breathing stopped at any time during the accident.

If the patient is conscious, he will probably be very frightened by the situation of being in hospital as the subject of a lot of investigations which he probably cannot understand fully. Many patients feel unnerved by being the centre of activity which they can neither contribute to nor control. There may be moments of frenetic activity during the immediate emergency admission, followed by seemingly endless, frustrating periods of waiting when it may seem that nothing is being done to 'make the patient better'. You can help the patient's emotional and physical state by remaining calm and reassuring. You should also remember that the unconscious patient may still be aware of his surroundings because he can hear and understand, even though he cannot see or speak, so you should take care to talk to the patient reassuringly, and not to say or do anything that might be alarming to him. The unconscious patient who has had a head injury may even be drawn back towards consciousness if you talk to him about familiar or favourite things.

It is important for relatives or companions to try to understand what is happening, partly to alleviate their own anxieties, and mainly in order to help the patient. You can help not only by being positively reassuring and avoiding adding to the patient's alarm, but also you can play a part in helping the patient's recovery. Although relatives should never interfere with the process of medical examination and treatment, you should be prepared, at the appropriate moment, to ask the relevant questions which will enable you to understand what has happened and what the outcome might be. You may only have limited opportunities for asking the medical staff questions, so it is often helpful to have written them down as you think of them; this can save time, and may prevent you from forgetting an important point.

You might want to ask some of these questions:

- What is wrong with the patient?
- How or why has it happened?
- Is he going to die?
- What treatment can you give?
- Can the patient recover to be the same as before?
- Can you predict how long the patient might need to stay in hospital?
- What can I do to help?

The doctor may not be able to answer all these questions straight away, as some of the answers may depend on the results of investigations and diagnostic tests. If so, the doctor will explain what tests are going to be done, and what information the tests should give.

Diagnostic tests

The doctor usually goes through the clinical examination after taking the patient's history. To test the patient's reflexes, the doctor uses a circular rubber-headed 'hammer' to tap against the tendons at the elbows, wrists, knees and ankles. Normally, each part responds to this tap with a slight jerk, but if the central nervous system is damaged, the jerk is exaggerated. A special test is to scratch the sharp end of the hammer handle along the soles of the patient's feet: normally, this makes the big toe curl downwards involuntarily, but the abnormal reaction caused by a stroke or head injury makes the big toe turn upwards while the toes spread out: this is called *Babinski's Sign*.

The patient's eyes are examined. If the patient is unconscious, the tests are repeated at regular intervals hourly or half-hourly. The conscious patient may only be tested once or twice. A light is shone into the patient's eyes, and the doctor notes whether the pupils narrow (constrict) in the bright light and open up (dilate) as the light is taken away. The doctor looks into the eyes through an ophthalmoscope to check whether there is any swelling pressing on the optic nerve. In a few cases, the doctor will notice that the eyes are affected by involuntary rapid flickering movements, called nystagmus.

Other parts of the face are also examined. In the unconscious patient, the doctor checks the position of the tongue. If the patient can co-operate, the doctor asks him to raise his eyebrows, open his eyes widely and close them tightly, smile, and close his mouth and make a chewing action, followed by swallowing. Then the doctor may ask the patient to open his mouth, so that the position and movements of the tongue can be checked. Occasionally, the patient's senses of taste and smell may also be tested. All of these tests, including those for the eyes, are checks on the cranial nerves, which pass directly out of the brain into the various parts of the face.

The doctor checks the patient's awareness and orientation in time and place by asking simple questions. If possible, tests are done on balance and movement, to show the extent to which they are undamaged or impaired. The doctor asks the patient to move his arm and leg, sit and stand, according to his abilities. Increasingly, these functional tests are done by the chartered physiotherapist as part of the assessment before starting the active rehabilitation programme.

The patient's blood pressure is monitored regularly. This may be done by special electrodes attached to the chest and wired to a television-like screen which also displays the pulse, a visual picture of the heart-beat, and the body temperature. Alternatively, blood pressure is measured using a sphygmomanometer: a small hand-pump is used to push air into a cuff attached to the patient's arm; the cuff is linked to a graduated mercury column, which rises as the air goes in, then falls as the air is slowly released by the doctor or nurse. Through a stethoscope held over the elbow, the examiner can hear when the heart pulse returns, and the corresponding levels of the mercury are recorded. This gives two readings: the upper level is called the systolic pressure, the lower is the diastolic pressure. If the blood pressure is higher than normal, the patient is said to be *hypertensive*; if it is abnormally low, the patient is *hypotensive*.

Blood tests are taken to show what is technically called the patient's blood picture. All the normal constituents of the blood, such as the red cells (corpuscles), platelets and haemoglobin are checked for signs of abnormal levels or activity. The doctors may only need a small syringe-full of blood to check all the important factors. If the patient is placed on anti-clotting drugs, for example Heparin or Warfarin, the effectiveness of the treatment is monitored at regular intervals by further blood tests, which may only involve a pinprick on the thumb.

Very occasionally, a lumbar puncture may be performed. The doctor puts a large needle into the spinal canal in the lower back in order to extract a little of the fluid which circulates around the spinal cord and through the brain (cerebrospinal fluid). The fluid, which is normally clear, is checked for the presence of blood.

The electrocardiogram (ECG) is a visual picture of the pattern of the patient's heart-beat. Electrodes on the chest, or on the wrists and ankles, are attached by leads to a machine called an electrocardiograph, which picks up electrical signals from the heart as it beats. This may be done once, as a routine test which takes only about five minutes, or it may be repeated at regular intervals. Patients in intensive care are usually on continuous electrocardiograph monitoring.

An angiogram is an x-ray taken of the arteries and veins after the patient has been given an injection, usually in the arm or neck, of a radio-opaque substance. The patient may be given a mild anaesthetic or muscle relaxant before the procedure. The radiologist watches as the x-ray shows the circulation of the dye through the patient's blood vessels, and he is able to pinpoint any areas of narrowing, constriction, blockage, widening or weakening. This would show, for instance, the exact site of a thrombus or aneurysm.

Computerized axial tomography, more familiarly known as a CAT scan, is a special type of x-ray which can show up where a blood clot lies, or where brain damage has occurred. The radiologist may enhance the picture by using a contrast medium, in which case the patient is given an injection before the scan is done.

Magnetic Resonance Imaging (MRI) is another diagnostic technique which uses computer technology to produce a 'picture' of the tissues. Instead of x-rays, magnetic fields are used to cause the emission of wavelengths from the brain, and these are amplified before being translated into a visual image by the computer.

The electroencephalogram (EEG) is a graph showing the rhythmical electrical activity of the brain. Electrodes placed round the patient's head are linked to a machine called an electroencephalograph. The test reveals trauma to the brain, and is done routinely in cases of head injury, but it may also be done for the stroke victim if the doctors feel there is a specific reason for it. If the patient's condition deteriorates, the EEG may be repeated at intervals. A totally non-responsive (flat) EEG is one of the proofs that the brain is dead.

Brain death and organ donation

Relatives may find themselves in the sad and difficult position of being told by the doctors that the patient has died after admission to hospital. This is technically termed 'brain death'. The doctors will have tried everything to save the patient's life, and they will only define the patient as brain dead if there is a complete absence of electrical activity in the brain as measured on the electroencephalogram; if the patient is totally unable to breathe by himself; if he has fixed, dilated pupils; and if he does not respond at all to painful or obnoxious stimuli. These tests are always done more than once, by more than one doctor, before the doctors finally conclude that the patient is brain dead.

The patient will look as if he is still alive, as his vital systems are being maintained on the life-support machine. However, once brain death has occurred and been confirmed, there is no hope that the patient might recover and live. At this stage the doctors will offer you the chance to pay last respects to the patient, and, if you wish, you can be present when the life-support machine is switched off. If the patient was carrying an Organ Donor Card, the doctors will ask you if you have any objections to the patient's wishes being carried out. If there was no Donor Card, the doctors may still ask you for permission to remove specific organs in order to save another patient's life. You are at liberty to refuse, or you may wish only to offer one organ rather than several. If you are uncertain, you may be offered, or may ask for, counselling. The patient's life-support machine will not be switched off until the question of organ donation has been decided: if any organ is to be donated from the patient's body, the life-support machine will remain on until after it has been removed.

The trauma of this situation is reduced, up to a point, when people carry Organ Donor Cards. If the victim has already foreseen that he would like to help another person, even after his own death, it makes the decision easier for his relatives, especially if he has already discussed with them the possibility of donating his organs in the case of unexpected death.

5
The Patient in the Hospital Ward

The rehabilitation team in hospital consists of physio-therapists, occupational therapists, speech therapists and possibly clinical psychologists. The physiotherapists and occupational therapists are likely to assess each new stroke or head-injured patient on the ward, and then decide between them on the patient's treatment regime. The doctor in charge of a patient usually decides whether the patient needs speech therapy or psychological treatment, and requests these practitioners to assess the patient and treat him according to their findings. The rehabilitation team works in close liaison with the doctors and nurses on the wards, as treatment has to be unified to be successful, and this depends on good communications between all the practitioners. Treatment facilities vary from hospital to hospital, and the amount of rehabilitation care a patient receives may depend on the availability of staff, but ideally, active treatment starts immediately the patient is stable following a stroke or head injury. All the treatment is done with sensitivity towards the patient: even if he cannot communicate verbally, any signs of distress tell the therapist that the treatment needs to be modified. He is treated gently, never harshly, as any physical or emotional upset is likely to lead to unwanted and uncontrollable spastic reactions which hinder the patient's ability to move successfully.

The unconscious patient

Nowadays, family and close friends are encouraged to visit the stroke or head-injured patient, even if he is unconscious when he is transferred to the ward. They can help him return to consciousness by talking gently to him, reading books and newspapers aloud, and perhaps playing tape recordings of his favourite music. Visitors are usually advised on how they can help. You may be encouraged to touch the patient, perhaps stroking the face, holding hands, or kissing him, as you might do normally. There is usually careful guidance on how much you should do on each occasion and how long you should stay, to avoid the risk of over-stimulating the patient, making him agitated, and perhaps pushing him further into unconsciousness.

The unconscious patient is nursed lying down in bed. It may be an ordinary hospital bed on high legs with wheels, or a mattress on the floor, to minimize the risk of the patient falling out of bed. Floor-level nursing is often chosen for the head-injured patient who is likely to be very restless. If the patient is expected to be unconscious for a long time, he may lie on an airflow bed, which is specially designed to minimize the pressure created by the patient's own body-weight. Everything that is done to and for the patient is done carefully, as incorrect handling provokes automatic reactions of increased spasticity throughout the patient's affected (hemiplegic) side. Some Area Health Authorities have 'statutory lifts', which all their nursing and paramedical staff are required to use as standard practice when they move a patient, to safeguard both patients and staff. While the nurses care for the routine daily needs of the patient, doctors usually come to examine the patient at regular intervals each day. The physiotherapist and occupational therapist are involved from an early stage. The therapist usually works with the nurses, helping to choose the best position for the patient, and advising on handling techniques. Positioning charts are used in specialist units, and sometimes on general wards. They record the way in which the patient is being handled, and serve as guidelines to ensure that all members of the treatment team move and position him in the same way.

Usually, the patient is kept on his side, and turned to the other side every two hours, to prevent pressure sores from forming where the body's skin lies in constant contact with the sheets. The patient's position in bed is carefully arranged: there are pillows under his head, which is placed in the neutral position, not bent forwards or backwards; if he is lying on the affected hemiplegic side, the hip is placed straight in line with the trunk, and the affected shoulder is put to lie slightly forward of the body; lying on the unaffected side, the hemiplegic leg is stretched straight slightly behind the trunk; in either case, there is a pillow under the upper-most arm and another between the patient's legs; most importantly, there is a pillow in front of the patient's stomach, to prevent him from falling forward, and to give him a feeling of contact, as he may not be able to feel the bed when he lies on his affected side, and this often gives the patient a frightening feeling of floating. The bed usually has cot sides to protect the patient from falling out of bed. If he is not restless, the cot side may be on one side of the bed only, behind the patient, to minimize the feeling of 'imprisonment behind bars'.

Whenever the patient is to be turned over, two nurses lift him carefully from behind to place him on his back, before lifting him to the side of the bed or sliding him over by pulling the under-sheet sideways. The patient is then rolled onto his side, and carefully repositioned with the pillows rearranged. The unconscious patient is tube-fed. A catheter, or tube connected to the bladder, collects the patient's urine. Faeces are collected on a special small sheet in the centre of the bed, or the patient wears nappies. The nurses wash the patient regularly, to prevent infections. They often apply special creams after a wash to help protect the skin against pressure sores. Mouth toilet is done with a toothbrush or small mouth hose. All the nursing care is performed very gently. Harsh movements round the mouth, for instance, can greatly increase the spasticity in the affected side of the body. When the patient suffers from a 'bite reflex', any stimulation in the mouth not only provokes increased spasticity, but also a violent clenching of the teeth, sometimes so hard that the teeth break. Head-injured patients are specially likely to suffer from this abnormal reaction, and the orthodontist usually provides a specially fitted tooth guard to prevent damage. The nurses and everyone else handling the patient explain all their actions, so that he is not subjected to sudden or possibly frightening handling.

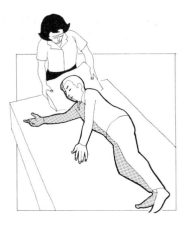
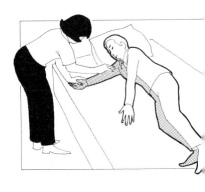
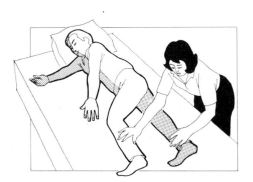
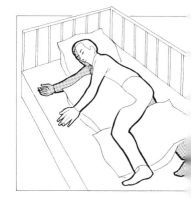

Positioning the unconscious patient in bed, lying on his hemiplegic side.

Washing

When the nurses wash the patient, the process of washing is considered to be part of the rehabilitation treatment. Even if the patient is unconscious, he is washed with care, in order not to stimulate his body badly and elicit the wrong body reactions. The unconscious patient is treated as though he is aware of what is going on, even though he gives no outward sign of this. The nurse aims to help the patient to keep in contact with his own body, physically. Although the nurse has to do the work of washing the patient, she moves the patient's hands to touch his own face and body, including his genitals. She also talks to the patient, explaining what she is doing at every stage. The speed at which the washing movements are performed is very important: if the movements are too fast, the patient's spasticity increases, and the nurse has to take care to avoid this.

The patient is not held in one position too long. Each part is moved gently before it is washed. This is specially important for mouth toilet, where the nurse has to handle the mouth and teeth extremely gently to avoid stimulating the bite reflex. When the arm is washed, the nurse moves it at the shoulder first, and similarly moves the hip before washing the leg. To wash the lower legs and feet, the nurse might place the feet in a bowl of water on the bed, with a plastic sheet or mackintosh under the bowl: she then sponges the legs down from the knees. Special care has to be taken when handling the feet, to avoid stimulating the reflexes which would send the patient into an automatic stiffening through his body. As the patient is turned over in bed, the nurse tells him which direction he is moving to, and asks him to follow the movement with his eyes. Sometimes this is the first outward indication that the patient can understand and is aware of his surroundings. When the nurse washes the patient's back, she continues to describe the sequence of what she is doing, and to involve the patient's hands in the parts he can reach easily.

Drying the patient is part of the same process of performing a practical task while making it into an education in self-awareness and awareness of the environment. The nurse takes care to dry the patient gently but thoroughly. She then applies creams, if necessary, to any pressure areas, or any skin parts which might be starting to look sore.

Physiotherapy treatment

Even if the patient is unconscious, he is likely to be given physiotherapy treatment. If he is still attached to a ventilator (life-support machine), he is treated in the Intensive Care Unit. If he is being nursed on the ward, he will probably be wheeled to the physiotherapy department on a trolley for his rehabilitation treatment. The unconscious patient may be flaccid or very spastic, with his muscles contorting him uncontrollably. The physiotherapist's aim is to try to promote some useful muscle activity against the effect of gravity, and this involves getting the patient into the upright position. The therapist explains all the actions and movements to the patient, and also asks him to co-operate. For the flaccid patient, the instructions are usually simple commands such as 'Hold!' or 'Stay!' to encourage any muscle activity which occurs. The spastic patient is instructed 'Let go!' or 'Don't push!' to dampen down unwanted muscle reactions. The physiotherapist takes care never to frighten the patient by unexpected movements. The speed of each action is geared to the patient's condition and responses, so that slower, larger range movements are used for the spastic patient than for the flaccid one.

For a first experience of standing, the unconscious patient

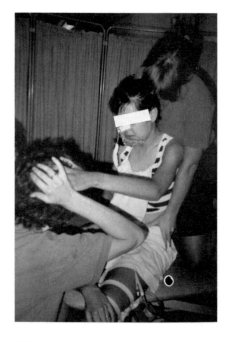

Treating the unconscious patient: the patient's position is carefully controlled, while the physiotherapists encourage awareness through touch.

is sometimes placed on a tilt table, a specially designed board to which the patient is strapped safely, in order to turn him gently into the upright position without any danger of falling. The disadvantage of the tilt table is that it is completely passive. The physiotherapist often prefers to try to evoke responses from the patient. She may start this by manœuvring him into the sitting position on the side of a treatment couch. She then stands behind the patient, controlling his head and trunk in order to create rhythmical movements by swaying his body gently forwards and backwards, and from side to side. The flaccid patient usually responds by beginning to straighten up. For the spastic patient, the movements are calculated to reduce the spastic responses, so that the patient begins to balance without abnormal distorting reactions against the supporting surface and the physiotherapist.

The next stage is for the patient to be helped to stand, and this is normally done with one physiotherapist standing on the couch behind the patient, while a second physiotherapist sits on a low stool in front of him. The therapists position the patient's pelvis and trunk so that he can be levered into the standing position without effort, and he is then supported and moved gently to transfer his weight from side to side, while the physiotherapist behind him supports his head in the correct position. Between them, the physiotherapists position the patient's pelvis and trunk to help overcome some of his involuntary spastic reactions, enabling him to stand securely, with good balance.

Another important part of the unconscious patient's rehabilitation is the desensitization of his mouth. Irritation of the mouth from suction and feeding tubes often causes severe spastic responses and leads to the bite reflex. For mouth treatment, the patient may be positioned lying on a foam wedge with his legs stretched apart. The physiotherapist sits by his hemiplegic side, supporting his head, gently moves his cheek in a massage-like motion, and then rubs his gums with a clean finger or toothbrush. Finally, the physiotherapist moves his tongue gently, with her finger, a toothbrush or a spatula. If the patient clamps his jaws as these movements take place, the physiotherapist tells him 'No!', and restarts the process, encouraging signs of awareness such as the patient pursing or smacking his lips. Encouraging the right responses and discouraging inappropriate reactions are a constant element of rehabilitation that has to be continued throughout the day. Everyone around the patient should say 'No!' if the patient clenches or grinds his teeth, or if he indulges in primitive reflex activities such as playing with his genitals.

The unconscious patient may spend only twenty minutes in the physiotherapy department, but he is more likely to be treated over one and a half hours. He returns to the ward for feeding and nursing care. Ideally, he receives rehabilitation treatment every day, including the weekends, and he may even be treated twice a day. In between treatments he is positioned carefully on his bed, or on his mattress, if he is being nursed on the floor, so that the improvements in regaining muscle control are not spoiled by allowing involuntary spastic reactions to take over when the patient is at rest. The treatment regime continues until the patient's condition changes.

The conscious patient

The patient who is conscious stays in bed only to rest or sleep. He usually needs help to move around in bed, because of poor balance and lack of co-ordination, so he is positioned by the nurses in order to minimize any spastic reactions. When he lies on his back, a foam wedge is placed under his shoulders and head to prevent his shoulder girdle from pressing back into the bed. He does not use the sloping back-rest attached to the bed-head, as this would make him slide down the bed into a poorly supported position. Lying on his side, he is positioned like the unconscious patient. If he is resting in bed, but not sleeping, he is usually placed on his hemiplegic side, so that he can reach for objects in front of him, or roll safely onto his back on his wedge pillow. In order to move, the patient is taught to lever himself by bending his unaffected arm and leg. He is not given a 'monkey bar' to pull himself with, because any major effort of this kind would inevitably increase his spasticity.

For much of the day the patient sits out of bed, as there is no reason for him to stay in bed all day, especially as doing

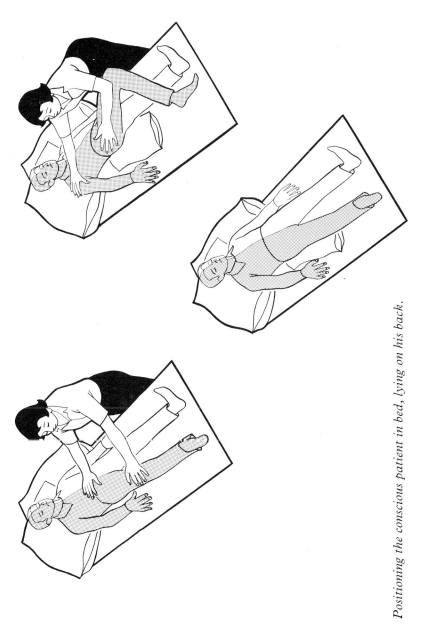

Positioning the conscious patient in bed, lying on his back.

so carries the risk of pressure sores, general body weakening and damage to the circulation. To get in and out of bed, he is initially lifted, so that he makes no effort at all, and therefore avoids provoking spastic reactions in his affected side. The lift can be done safely by one nurse. The patient lies on his side with his hands gently clasped together and his arms held forward. The nurse stands very close in front of him, supports his head, guides his hip-bone downwards and levers his body gently upwards. She then manoeuvres him forwards by pulling each side of his seat forwards in turn. She asks the patient to rest his head on her shoulder away from the chair they are aiming at. She presses her thighs against the patient's knees, pulls his pelvis forwards, and swivels so that the patient lands gently into his chair. She does not handle the affected shoulder if possible, to avoid causing pain in the joint, and to minimize the risk of wrenching it out of its socket.

When the patient is out of bed, he may sit in a wheelchair or an upright chair. The wheelchair is chosen if the patient needs to be transported to the toilet or other parts of the hospital at frequent intervals. If the patient is capable of transporting himself in a wheelchair, he is usually issued with an electric motorized chair, rather than one with single side wheel control, as the effort of working the latter would tend to increase spastic reactions in the hemiplegic side. The wheelchair is specially chosen, usually by the physiotherapist or occupational therapist, to suit the patient. It has a specially moulded back support, and a seat cushion to relieve pressure and prevent the patient from sagging into a bent position. It has two foot plates, on which the patient's feet are placed flat. They are at the right height to hold the patient's knees slightly downwards in relation to his hips. A flat tray-table is fixed to the front of the wheelchair, with comfortable space left in front of the patient's stomach, so that he can move around slightly in the chair. Ideally, the table is perspex, so that the patient can see his feet and correct the affected foot if it slips off the foot-plate. (He may need to ask the nurse to replace his foot in the right position.) He sits with both arms resting on the table.

The patient is not left to sit in the wheelchair for long periods, as he cannot change position to any extent, so the

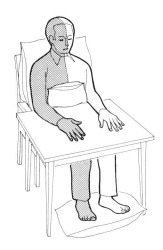

Sitting correctly.

wheelchair becomes uncomfortable after a while. An upright chair is chosen according to the same principles as a wheelchair. The patient sits with most of the thigh length supported, knees slightly below hip level, and feet flat on the floor or cushioned on a pillow. The chair back supports the patient up to shoulder level, but not up to head level, in case the patient tends to press back against it, producing spastic reactions. The chair has arms, but the patient does not rest the hemiplegic arm on the side, as it would tend to slip off. A pillow is placed on the patient's lap to support his stomach and help prevent him from falling forwards, and his affected arm rests in front of him on the pillow where he can see and control it.

The patient may sit out in his chair for about three hours at a time. The chair may be placed at a long table, so that groups of patients can socialize. If not, the patient may have a small but solid table placed in front of his chair, or alternatively he might sit by the side of his bed with the objects he needs during the day on the bed, within easy reach of his unaffected arm.

Going to the toilet

When he needs to go to the toilet, the patient is transported by wheelchair, if the ward toilets are designed to the correct specifications for patients who cannot walk. Bed-pans are avoided if at all possible, as they are awkward to use, and can therefore provoke severe spastic reactions throughout the patient's body. The nurse helps the patient transfer from the wheelchair onto the toilet, taking care to avoid any stress or effort on the patient's part, to avoid an increase in spasticity. If the toilets are not suitable for wheelchair access, the nurse brings a commode (portable toilet) into the patient's cubicle and draws the curtains round the cubicle. If the patient's sitting balance is poor, the nurse stays with him while he is on the toilet, otherwise she leaves him in privacy. Whether on the commode or in the toilet, the patient usually has a call-button to summon the nurse when he has finished, or in case he gets into difficulties.

Washing

If he is conscious, the patient is expected to take part in the washing procedures; he is not simply washed passively just to make sure that he is clean. The nurse is not just cleansing the patient, but re-educating him to wash himself. Before starting, the nurse has to assess what balance problems he has, if any, first when he is sitting down, then standing up, if he can stand. Nurses would probably ask the physiotherapists for this information, but specially trained stroke care nurses would be able to make these judgements for themselves. The nurse also has to be aware of any perceptual problems the patient might have. A routine is established, so that the patient gets to a certain method of practising washing. If different nurses handle the patient and wash him, they liaise among themselves in order to keep to a set routine, to avoid confusing the patient. The nurses may ask you, the carer, what type of soap and shaving foam the patient normally uses, in order to remind him that washing is a familiar everyday activity.

The patient is taken to the bathroom, if possible, to make him aware of the realistic context for washing. All the materials needed, such as soap, flannels and towels, are prepared beforehand, and placed around the patient at different angles, to encourage him to move in different directions. The patient may sit in his wheelchair in front of the basin, and watch himself in a mirror. The nurse may ask him to put the plug in, turn on the taps and fill the basin, guiding him if he is uncertain. She then asks him to pick up the soap, and start to wash his face. If he cannot yet perform these actions because of perceptual problems and failure to recognize what soap is or where his face is, the nurse helps him through the sequence, reinforcing her verbal instructions by helping the patient to touch the soap and then his face. She describes each part of the face as the patient touches it, and helps him to orientate downwards from forehead to chin, and sideways between left and right, not forgetting the ears.

Washing then proceeds down the body: the patient starts washing his chest in the centre, working round to either side systematically, under the nurse's guidance. The nurse moves around him rather than staying on one side only, and helps him to wash from his back, round under his armpits, and then down the arms to his wrists and hands. On the hemiplegic side, she takes care to avoid stimulating the grasp reflex in the hand as she and the patient wash it. When the patient washes his abdomen, she encourages him to feel the whole line of his waist. If he can, he uses both hands for the washing movements for his trunk, although the hemiplegic hand may need careful support and guidance. As the patient washes and dries himself sitting down, the nurse encourages balanced trunk movements, and watches carefully to make sure that the patient's spasticity is not increased by his efforts. If this happens, she gives the patient a rest, and then gives him more help in completing the task, perhaps even doing it all gently herself. If she applies talcum powder or cream to his skin, the nurse describes what she is doing, and asks the patient to help, if possible. She also describes what the skin should feel as the cream or powder touches it, to help the patient remember normal skin sensations.

If the patient can stand up, his pelvic region is washed as he stands, but if this is too difficult, he washes his lower body lying down on the bed, with protective sheeting underneath him. At all stages of the washing process, the nurse takes care to avoid over-tiring the patient, or increasing his spasticity.

When she repeats the sequence the next day, whether she goes through washing the whole body or only part of it, she tries to repeat the exact order she has followed previously, to help reinforce the patient's memory of what he is doing. If he is too tired on some days to take much active part in it, the nurse does more of the work herself, but still describes the actions to the patient so that he is involved in it and does not just let himself be handled passively.

For a first experience of sitting in the bath, the patient may be lifted in with a special overhead hoist. If the patient progresses well enough, he may be taught to get into the bath normally before he leaves hospital, although this will not be done if it is so difficult for him that it increases his spasticity.

Eating and drinking

Most hemiplegic patients can eat and drink normally, so meals are just a routine part of the day's activities. They may be on a special diet, worked out by the dietician, to control weight, diabetes or blood pressure. If the patient was accustomed to drinking a lot of alcohol each day before his stroke or accident, the doctors may prescribe an alcohol replacement, although drinking any real alcohol after the stroke or head injury is strongly discouraged. A chart of food and fluid intake may be kept by the nursing staff, so everything the patient eats and drinks is accurately recorded, usually together with a chart of urine output and bowel movements. Patients who have been tube-fed during a long period of unconsciousness may have to relearn how to eat, simply because of lack of practice. Feeding through the nasogastric tube may continue while the patient learns to eat normally again.

Some patients can manage to eat, but only with difficulty, because of loss of control over one side of the face (facial palsy or facial dysfunction). The problem usually lies in chewing and moving the food round the mouth ready for swallowing, although actually taking the food into the mouth, biting and swallowing can be done normally. Hemiplegic patients can have great and sometimes permanent problems eating. Head-injured patients are specially likely to suffer from difficulties in eating and swallowing. If they cannot feel the food inside their mouths, they have to make a conscious effort to remember to swallow it down after chewing. Some have difficulty closing their lips, so they tend to drool, and food falls out of their mouths.

Eating difficulties make mealtimes an important part of the patient's therapy, as recovering the ability to eat normally is an important part of returning to normal life. It is also important because the patient who cannot co-ordinate his eating actions is in danger of spluttering on his food, drawing it into the trachea and causing pneumonia. The physiotherapist, occupational therapist or speech therapist may perform the tasks of reteaching normal eating. One of these practitioners may take on sole responsibility for this aspect of the patient's rehabilitation, or they may take it in turns by mutual agreement. The therapist teaches the patient who drools to dab his mouth clean, and to close his lips gently with his hand. The nurses remind him to do this at frequent intervals, so that the skin and muscles do not remain permanently over-stretched. Movements of the mouth, lip and tongue are gradually retaught, using different types of food.

The dietician usually sets out the patient's food programme in conjunction with the therapist, at first choosing foods which are easy to bite, chew and swallow, and then gradually introducing more difficult foods. Different tastes stimulate tongue movements, so flavourings are chosen with care. Lightly cooked vegetables may be the first food offered to the patient, followed by combinations of foods, such as fruit yoghurt on celery and vegetables in different sauces. Meat, cut up by the therapist, comes at a later stage, if the patient is not vegetarian. Then chunks of food of different consistency are introduced, such as goujons, fish fingers and pieces of fruit. In order to teach the patient eating control, the therapist starts by supporting his head and face. She then offers a piece of food, holding it with light pressure against the patient's teeth. She tells him when to bite, and helps him to swallow by manipulating his tongue from under his chin at the right moment. This helps both his eating action and his timing of it. This process is repeated each meal time with the different types of food until the patient can feed himself.

Fluids and soft foods, such as minced meat and mashed potatoes, are among the hardest substances to swallow. Even

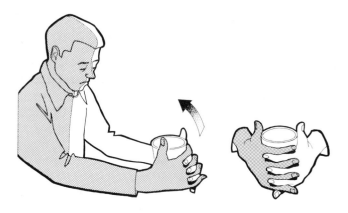

The clasp grip for holding a cup or glass.

in the earliest stages, fluids are presented to the patient in a cup or glass. A spout beaker is not used, because it does not help the patient to relearn swallowing, and it makes it dangerously easy to pour liquid down his throat and into his lungs. To help the patient swallow correctly, the therapist supports his head while he is sitting up straight. The cup is held with light pressure against the patient's lower lip. If possible, the patient holds both hands round the cup, although the therapist supports the cup's weight. The therapist then shows the patient how to tip the cup back, rather than tipping his head back. If his tongue thrusts forward as the fluid enters his mouth, it has to be corrected. As the fluid goes into the patient's mouth, the therapist puts a little downward pressure on his upper lip, and then helps the swallowing action by pressurizing the tongue from under his chin. Thick fluids such as soups and yoghurt are the easiest to drink, while water is the hardest, so the patient progresses gradually from one to the other.

Dressing

Dressing is a practical activity which is also part of the rehabilitation retraining regime. The patient is not expected to learn quickly how to dress himself unaided, because the process is even more complicated than walking. Neither do the nurses or therapists dress him passively, without asking him to co-operate and learn. In order to dress, the patient has to practise balancing, first of all sitting down, later standing up; he has to distinguish between left and right; and he has to work out where each part of his clothing fits on to his body. Therefore, dressing is not just a physical task but an exercise in self-awareness and awareness of the environment which is specially important for patients with perceptual difficulties. It is taken stage by stage, and each day the patient practises what he has learned on previous days, and learns new movements when he is ready. Ideally, the occupational therapist or physiotherapist works with the nurses first thing in the morning to help the patient to dress. The occupational therapist may repeat some of the dressing training in detail later in the day in the occupational therapy department.

Suitable clothing is chosen, preferably a loose-fitting tracksuit with a jacket top for male and female alike, and carers are usually asked to bring in the patient's own clothes from home. Because he must avoid making unnecessary effort, in order to control his spasticity, the patient is guided through each stage of dressing, and helped where necessary. For instance, he may be able to put his hemiplegic arm into his sleeve without trouble, but he may not be able to balance and lean forward safely enough to put on his trousers by himself, so the therapist and/or nurse helps. Coping with trousers is used as practice in sitting and leaning forward to place the trousers by his feet, but the therapist then does the work of pulling up the trousers. If the patient has just progressed to the stage of standing up from a chair, the therapist pulls up the trousers while the patient concentrates on balancing. When the patient can stand up confidently with the therapist's help, he may pull up his own trousers while the therapist helps him to maintain his balance. If he has recovered some use in his hemiplegic arm, he uses both hands together on the trousers. Every aspect of relearning dressing is carefully graded to the individual patient's ability.

Safe shoes are essential, and slippers are definitely dangerous, so the patient may be kept barefoot until appropriate shoes are brought in for him. As the patient's hemiplegic foot may be swollen, he may need a slightly larger size in shoes than usual, and he may be given special support stockings to wear to help his circulation. His hemiplegic ankle may be unstable, tending to twist on itself, so the therapist may recommend boots with velcro fastenings, or may supply him with a rigid stirrup-shaped ankle support of the kind used for sprained ankles. Training shoes, again with velcro fastenings, are very practical, although the patient may prefer stouter leather lace-up shoes. Any laces should be elastic, for easy management with one hand. Shoe soles should not be too thick or rigid, as the patient needs to feel the floor underfoot when he is trying to balance standing up. If the patient cannot lean forward safely, the nurse or therapist puts his shoes on for him. When he has learned to sit and lean forward, he is taught to lift his hemiplegic leg up across the other with his hand, in order to put his shoe on. He also puts his shoe on his unaffected leg by bringing that leg over the hemiplegic leg, so that he learns symmetrical patterns of movement.

Physiotherapy treatment

Usually in the morning, after breakfast, the patient is taken by wheelchair to the physiotherapy department for rehabilitation. If his blood pressure is unstable following the stroke, or if there is some other medical reason why he cannot be taken to the department, he is kept on the ward, but this phase usually only lasts a few days. While some rehabilitation treatment can be done on the ward, it is best done in the physiotherapy and occupational therapy departments, where there is adequate space and equipment such as adjustable couches (treatment plinths). The patient may be apprehensive about rehabilitation, so, if possible, the need for it is carefully explained, and everything that will happen to the patient is described in detail, even if the patient has language difficulties and may not understand everything. Friends and relatives can help by repeating the explanation that rehabilitation is the only method through which the patient can get better. The patient with severe perceptual problems and language difficulties may not be helped by verbal explanations: in this case the physiotherapist guides the patient through the required actions, giving very simple commands at the same time.

In the physiotherapy department, the emphasis is on

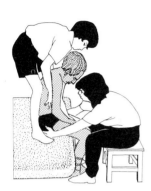

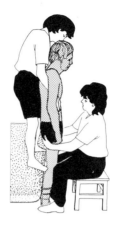

The inactive patient in a flexed posture: he has no balance in his trunk, so he cannot sit upright.

The patient brought into the standing position, to encourage extension activity.

physical recovery. Standing is a vital element in rehabilitation, as good balance when standing up is the basis for independent mobility. The patient has to learn to sit up safely, and to stand up from sitting and vice versa. For the flaccid patient, the priority is to prevent the natural tendency to overuse the unaffected side, as this makes stable balance impossible. The physiotherapist concentrates on promoting trunk movements to equalize the work done by both the right and left sides of the body. When the patient is standing up, the physiotherapist helps him learn how to shift his weight over the hemiplegic side and then recover his balance to stand straight again. The techniques for teaching sitting and standing balance are different for the spastic patient, who has to learn how to reduce unwanted muscle activity before he can make effective movements. The therapist prepares the spastic patient for standing by moving him slowly in different directions in gentle rhythmical patterns, while the patient remains seated and makes no effort at all until the spastic reactions are controlled. Then the therapist helps the patient to stand up and he practises balancing and transferring his weight from one foot to the other. The patient also practises movements involving the affected arm, and learns how to lie down from the sitting position, and then to sit up from the lying position. All these movements are very complicated, and the patient has to learn how to do them in easy, controlled stages.

Physiotherapy treatment can last for up to one and a half hours, and the patient may then return to the ward to have lunch and rest. Part of the day may be spent in the occupational therapy department, where the active movements the patient is relearning may be put to use in functional activities such as dressing, eating and drinking, or performing tasks designed to improve self-awareness and spatial awareness. In the very early stages, for instance, the patient may do children's jigsaw puzzles to help him recognize shapes and visual images; he may do reading and writing exercises; and he may relearn basic daily tasks such as how to tell the time. The patient with speech and understanding difficulties usually also attends the speech therapy department for individual training in recognizing and using words, and, where necessary, in feeding and swallowing.

As soon as possible, the patient is encouraged to walk between the different departments in the hospital, although he may still need a wheelchair for longer distances, or when he gets tired.

How you can help when you visit the patient in hospital

- Be reassuring at all times. The patient will inevitably be depressed and frustrated following a stroke or head injury. Avoid giving him bad news. If possible, tell him stories you know will please and entertain him, perhaps about his family and friends, or anecdotes from the newspapers. Talk to him, even if he cannot respond, but watch for signs that he is getting distressed by what you say, or tired.

- Try to help him understand what is going on, particularly in relation to his rehabilitation treatment, as it is vital for him to realize that rehabilitation is the only method of

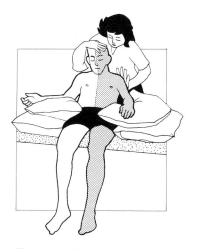 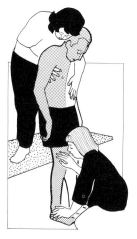

Teaching the patient to control forward movements using his trunk, shoulders and head: the first stage towards sitting up without support.

Working to desensitize the positive supporting reaction in the foot, so that the patient can stand safely.

treatment which will make him better and prevent him from getting worse.

- Bring in appropriate shoes and clothing, taking the therapists' and nurses' advice as to what is needed.

- Do not bring the patient cigarettes or alcohol, unless the doctors have given specific permission for him to have them.

- Remember that the patient may be on a special diet, or he may have swallowing difficulties, so check with the doctors, nurses or therapists whether the patient can have food such as biscuits or fruit, or soft drinks, before bringing these as gifts.

- If the patient can read, bring him newspapers and books. He may need big books with large print. If he cannot cope with a whole newspaper, because he cannot concentrate for long enough, he may enjoy articles cut out and stuck onto plain paper. If he cannot read, he may still enjoy listening to stories, even if he has speech and understanding difficulties, so you can read to him or bring him tapes to play.

- Calming music is very therapeutic. To avoid disturbing other patients, a personal stereo cassette player is suitable. Stereo headphones are preferable to a single earpiece, as they make the patient aware of both sides of his head. If the patient cannot manage to work the player by himself, you can listen to the music with him at visiting times, if you have a player with two headphone sockets.

- Some games and puzzles can be good mental and physical exercises for the patient, so you can ask the therapists which would be the most appropriate to bring in for him. If the patient gets frustrated with a task, teach him to leave it and come back to it fresh later, rather than persevering without success, or leaving it completely.

- You should ask the therapists to show you how to position the patient, so that you can help in making correct positioning a continuous process. The patient may slip down in his chair during your visit, for instance, or his hemiplegic hand may drop down, so you should know how to replace him in good posture without any risk of harming him. If you are willing, the therapists may show you how to help the patient to stand up and sit down, and how to help his eating if he has difficulties.

- A daily diary is a useful record of the patient's progress, and a valuable mental exercise for him. If he can speak but not write, you can write the diary for him as a record of his comments and feelings. If he cannot speak, you can note down any improvements you see day by day. In the later stages of recovery, it can be both reassuring and encouraging to remember how the patient was immediately after the stroke or head injury.

Weekend leave and discharge from hospital

As the patient's rehabilitation progresses, he is usually allowed home for weekends, partly to give him increased motivation to return to normal life, and partly to get him and his family used to coping in home surroundings. The carer is taught how to handle the patient. You may have to learn how to transfer or lift him, and how to position him in a chair or in bed. You will not only watch these techniques being done by the therapists, but will practise them under the therapists' guidance before the first weekend leave takes place. If several members of the family are to be involved in caring for the patient, they will all be taught the correct handling techniques, so that everyone can be reasonably confident of coping. Some rehabilitation units have little flats or bed-sitting rooms, where patients, either alone or with their carers, can practise independent living before their first trip home. This has several advantages: professional help is close at hand, if needed, and the patient can concentrate on what he has to do, without the distraction of familiar people and objects which might tire or distress him.

The carer is carefully instructed in what the patient should and should not be allowed to do. He has to be stopped from trying to do too much, and especially from trying to walk around, if he is not yet safe on his feet. On the other hand, he should be encouraged to join in his home or family life as much as possible, especially if he feels despondent and helpless at returning to his home surroundings when he is not well enough to do the things he did previously. The patient's stress has to be kept to a minimum: you have to remember that he will probably be elated at the thought of visiting his home, but at the same time he is likely to be apprehensive. He is very likely to find the experience tiring, if not exhausting. You have to try to balance his activities to make the experience as positive as possible. Visitors should be carefully controlled, so that they do not overwhelm the patient. You should try to invite only those people who are likely to have a good effect on the patient's spirits. Careful planning and counselling are needed to make it possible for the patient to enjoy his weekend leave without getting depressed or over-tired.

Weekend leave is an important step towards the patient's discharge from hospital. It may start with the patient going home for a single night, and then extend to the whole weekend when the patient is ready. Even a patient who has no one to look after him at home may go home on weekend leave, and the rehabilitation team will be 'on call' for him, in case he gets into difficulties. The district nurse or the 'meals on wheels' service may be asked to call in on him in the course of the weekend, to make sure he is all right.

The patient's stay in hospital may last from about eight weeks up to several months, depending on the severity of the stroke or head injury. The head-injured patient is more likely to need a prolonged hospital stay. The patient is discharged from hospital when he has reached a satisfactory stage of rehabilitation, which ideally is complete independence in walking and looking after himself. In practice, he is likely to need a measure of care. By the time he is discharged from hospital, he may still need a wheelchair if he is unable to walk safely unaided, or he may be walking with the help of a high stick. He may have recovered the use of his arm, but he is more likely to have some impairment in it, and he may even not be able to use it at all. His ability to manage living at home is assessed by members of the rehabilitation team, and their report is an important factor in deciding when he is ready to be discharged from hospital, and what sort of back-up services he is likely to need through his general practitioner and from the social services. Some patients may continue to attend the hospital for out-patient physiotherapy treatment. Most patients are recalled to the hospital at regular intervals for medical review, so that the doctors can check on their progress. This monitoring may continue for several years after the patient's stroke.

6
The Patient at Home

The professional support team

Following a stroke, the patient may be kept at home, rather than being admitted to hospital. This does not happen if there is any fear that the patient cannot cope, or if there is no one to look after him. Home care for the stroke patient may be chosen because the patient's doctor feels that the necessary rehabilitation can be done at home, or might be best done at home; the patient may be more comfortable, and therefore more co-operative to treatment if he remains among familiar surroundings; he might be liable to excessive stress if parted from his close family, friends or a beloved pet; or it may be a temporary situation, in which the patient is waiting for a bed in a specialist rehabilitation unit to become available.

Head-injured patients are normally admitted to hospital and kept there until it is certain that they are fully fit to return home. Like the stroke patient who has received hospital treatment, the head-injured patient may still be fairly disabled at the time he is discharged. In all cases, the general practitioner continues to monitor the patient's condition, prescribing any necessary drugs, such as those needed to control high blood pressure. Most importantly, he acts as the co-ordinator for the support services which the patient will need. The team involved in the care of the patient at home includes the district nurse, the community chartered physiotherapist, the occupational therapist and the social worker. If necessary, a speech therapist may be called on as well.

The *district nurse* is attached to the general practitioner surgery or health centre. She may be specially trained in some aspects of stroke care, so that she has the title of *stroke care nurse*. She is responsible for helping the patient and carers in daily tasks such as washing, bathing and going to the toilet. Where possible, she will help teach the patient

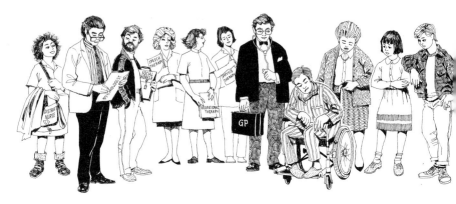

The rehabilitation team.

how to cope with these needs independently. Where necessary, she will supply useful items such as a wedge support, disposable sheets and incontinence pads. She advises on skin care, particularly in relation to avoiding pressure sores, and may supply sheepskin heel muffs to protect the feet, and sheepskin squares for the patient to sit or lie on. The district nurse usually comes to see the patient in the mornings, to help him get out of bed and wash. The patient who cannot sit up may start by washing in bed, with the nurse guiding him, so that he does not risk over-balancing and falling. As his condition improves, he gradually starts to wash while sitting, and later learns to get in and out of the bath. The nurse may also come back in the evening, especially in the beginning, in order to help the patient with medicines, such as insulin injections for diabetes, and to position him correctly in bed. It is essential for the carer to learn how to position the patient properly, so part of the district nurse's task is to teach the carer how to do this.

The *community physiotherapist* is part of the district physiotherapy service organized at the major local hospital, and the general practitioner has direct access to the service. The physiotherapist liaises with the hospital when the patient is due to be discharged, if he has been an in-patient. Her role may be restricted to advising the carers on how to treat the patient, and she may only visit the family once. Ideally, the community physiotherapist takes on the wider responsibility of not only teaching the carers, but also assessing and treating the patient's particular problems through a progressive rehabilitation programme. She may come to see the patient every day, usually excluding weekends. Having assessed the nature and extent of the patient's problems, she explains to the patient and his carers how the patient's physical recovery will happen. She sets out the details of how she feels the patient should be handled, so that the carers and everyone else involved will all help him to move in the same way. Day by day, she will give the patient an active treatment session through which he gradually relearns how to move on his own.

The *occupational therapist* in the community is normally employed by the social services department, and the initial contact is usually made by the general practitioner. The occupational therapist's main role is to assess the patient's physical needs, and provide appropriate equipment to make daily life easier for both patient and carer, so that they do not expend unnecessary energy on functional tasks which would make the patient's condition worse, and possibly harm the carer too. The occupational therapist might provide such items as a commode, blocks to raise the height of the bed, a suitable chair and possibly a wheelchair. The occupational therapist's role usually includes advising on suitable types of clothing for the patient, partly to make dressing simple and practical, and also so that the clothing chosen is helpful in the process through which the patient relearns to dress himself. The community occupational therapist also assesses whether the patient has any perceptual problems, such as an inability to recognize left and right, or total lack of awareness of the affected side of his body. These difficulties have to be explained to the carer, as they can be hard to understand. The occupational therapist plans suitable activities through which the carer can help the patient to overcome these perceptual problems.

The *social worker* might be called in by the general practitioner, district nurse, physiotherapist or the carer. The social worker is not usually involved in the early stages following the patient's stroke, but may be called in later if the patient is fairly severely disabled, or is an old person likely to need long-term support at home. In a sense, the social worker is responsible for the emotional and material well-being of the patient. There may be financial problems arising from the patient's illness, and the social worker can help in obtaining the benefit payments available from the State for patients and their carers, called the *attendance allowance*. The carer may be under too much stress, both physically and mentally, to cope with paperwork relating to such matters as the patient's sick pay from work, relevant insurance claims, or simply organizing payment of the normal household bills. The social worker can give practical help and advice on all these tasks. The patient and carer might also need a home help to clean the house or flat, or the social worker may call in 'care assistants', who are trained in very basic nursing skills, if the patient is too heavy for the carer to handle and move about alone. When there are problems in providing adequate meals for the patient, the social worker may bring in the 'meals on wheels' service. In a few cases, the social worker might have to make provision for young children to be given temporary care away from home, for instance if the patient is a single parent without any relatives who could care for the children. Similarly, pets such as dogs, cats or budgerigars have to be provided for, if it is not practical for anyone to look after them while the patient cannot.

Organizing the patient's living area

The patient needs space to move or be moved around in, and the home is organized accordingly. If the patient is moving around in a wheelchair, some furniture may have to be removed from his room to allow enough space for manoeuvring. The detailed arrangements vary according to the type of living accommodation the patient is in, but, if possible, everything is arranged so that the patient, carer, relatives, professional staff and visiting friends all move around without danger to themselves or the household furniture and decorations.

One priority is access to the toilet, or alternative toilet arrangements. In most cases, at least in the early stages, the patient needs help when transferring onto a commode or toilet, so there also has to be space for the carer. If the patient lives in a house with a downstairs toilet, a downstairs room may need to be turned into a bed-sitting room for him. If access to the toilet is difficult, perhaps because it has steps, or the room is too small for a wheelchair and the carer to manoeuvre in, he may have to be provided with a commode. Sometimes a commode is needed anyway for night-time use, although the patient can manage to use the toilet when he is fully awake and can plan the visit. Washing facilities are another priority, although in the early stages the patient might be washed in his room, as though he were in hospital.

For convenience, the patient's room is usually arranged as a bed-sitting room, if there is enough space. However, he should be taken out of his room at least occasionally, if at all possible, if only to avoid claustrophobia. It may be feasible for him to move into a separate sitting room for day-time activities, if the access is not difficult. Special care must be taken to ensure that the environment is safe for the patient to move about in. The floor must not be slippery, nor should there be loose rugs lying on it. The furniture should be arranged to allow free passage, and it is probably wise not to have breakable ornaments or glass-fronted cabinets in the areas where the patient will be.

At least at first, sharing a double bed is unlikely to be comfortable or practical for either patient or carer. If this was the sleeping arrangement prior to the patient's illness, the family may have to supply a fairly wide single bed for the patient, or the carer might sleep in a separate bed, leaving the normal conjugal bed to the patient. The bed should be as wide as space permits. It should be alongside the wall, or about one foot away from the wall to allow space for the carer, in case she needs to help the patient from that side. The head of the bed should be against a wall, or should have a head-board. When the patient is lying on his back, his hemiplegic side should be away from the side wall. The bed height should allow the patient to touch the floor with his feet when he sits on the side on the bed, although his hips should be slightly above the level of his knees. Most household beds need raising onto secure blocks to achieve this. On no account should the bed have wheels. It should be reasonably firm, but not too hard. A wooden board between the mattress and a sprung divan base is an acceptable alternative to a sprung mattress on a slatted wooden base. When the patient is in bed, he usually uses up to three pillows plus a wedge cushion support for his head and shoulders, to counteract spasticity (p. 49). His hemiplegic hip may be supported on a folded towel for the same reason, and he needs sheepskin muffs to protect his heels from pressure sores. A duvet is more practical than sheets, blankets and eiderdown, although the patient may prefer them if they are what he is used to.

The patient's chair and table are chosen according to the principles already described (p. 51). They are positioned so that the patient can get to and from the chair without too much effort. The table has to be solid enough not to give way when the patient rests on it, and it should be big enough to hold all the things the patient needs when he is out of bed. However, as the table has to be moved out of the way whenever the patient gets up, it should not be too heavy, or have too many items on it at one time. It is preferable to keep the table clear of objects other than those actually in use, while a sideboard within reach of the patient is used to hold the items which will be needed later. If the patient watches television, it should be positioned so that he is sitting straight to see it: he should not have to turn his head, or bend or crick his neck. Always check to make sure that electrical wires attached to the television or any other appliances, such as reading lamps, are well secured, so that they cannot trip people up.

Hemiplegic patients feel the cold, so extra home heating may be required. In houses where only the ground floor is centrally heated, the patient may not feel comfortable in the upstairs area, so if this is where he is to be, for other practical reasons, he will need heaters in his room, or the central heating system should be extended. If this creates financial hardship, the social worker may be able to help obtain grants to assist with the extra heating costs. Even in a centrally heated home, the patient may still feel the cold, so he may need to be dressed warmly, and wear thermal socks. He may even need to use a blanket over his legs when he is sitting in his chair. On no account should he use a hot water bottle, as it is likely to scald his skin, especially on his hemiplegic side.

While the patient should be kept warm, his room should also be properly ventilated, especially if he is in it all the time. If there is no other system of air-conditioning, and the window cannot be open all the time because of draughts or security, it should at least be opened once or twice a day for a spell.

Helping the patient to move around

Independence has to be achieved in stages. You and the patient may be anxious for him to be independent, but he should not try to move about or do things alone before he is ready. Both of you may also be keen for him to do 'exercises' to improve his physical condition. However, his 'homework' is strictly limited by the progress he has achieved during his rehabilitation treatment (p. 134). Until he can hold himself safely in the correct positions without increasing his spasticity when he is lying down, sitting, standing, or walking, he has to be helped to move in every situation. You have to be very aware of the patient's physical limitations in relation to his spasticity, in order to prevent him from trying to do more than he can, which would inevitably make his situation worse.

Getting the patient out of bed onto a chair, wheelchair or commode involves a *lift* or a *transfer*. With a lift, the carer takes control of the patient's full weight, so that he makes no effort in the manoeuvre, even when his feet are on the floor and he is effectively standing up. In a transfer the patient does as much as he can under instruction and with help from the carer, or he is able to transfer himself.

The patient is lifted if he has not recovered his ability to balance, that is, if he tends to topple and fall backwards and towards his hemiplegic side when he tries to sit or stand up without any support. In this case, the district nurse or physiotherapist will teach the carer how to lift the patient safely, and the lift must be used every time the patient needs to get out of bed or up from his chair. The point of using a lift is to prevent the patient from making any effort at all, so that he does not increase his spasticity by trying to achieve movements he is not yet capable of making successfully. There are several methods of lifting patients. They have been devised to place minimum strain on the lifter and her back, while ensuring that the patient is not at risk of falling or being dropped. Before the patient is moved, everything has to be arranged and ready. The chair or commode has to be correctly positioned, for instance, and firmly secured to prevent it from slipping away as the patient is moved. The wheelchair has both brakes on once it is in position. The patient's clothing should also be checked, so that there is no loose flapping material to get in the way.

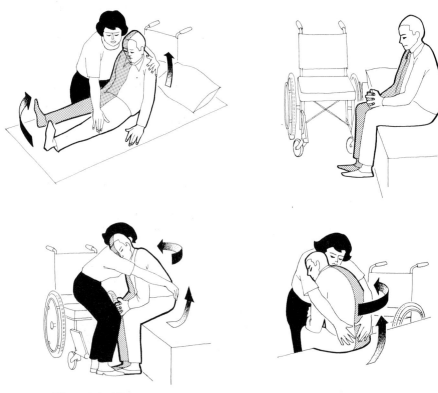

The pelvic lift.

One commonly used lifting method is the *pelvic lift*. To get out of bed, for instance, the patient is turned onto his side or lifted and then brought into the sitting position on the side of the bed. The carer gently levers him forwards by placing her hands behind his seat and swivelling his hips sideways and forwards. His feet should be flat on the floor. If he is moving to a wheelchair with a removable arm, it is placed at right angles to the bed, and his feet remain level with each other. If he is being moved onto a chair with fixed arms, the chair is placed at an angle of about 45° to the bed, and the patient's foot which is nearer the chair is placed slightly forwards relative to the other. The carer then asks the patient to clasp his hands together, and helps him to do this. He holds his hands passively forwards, and places his head on the carer's shoulder, on the side away from the chair. The carer stands with her legs on either side of the patient's knees, places her hands under the patient's seat, pulls his body-weight forward and in one movement lifts his pelvis and pivots him so that he sits down onto the chair.

The pelvic lift can also be used to move the patient from a wheelchair to a chair, or vice versa. Both chairs are placed securely, with the free chair at a slight angle to where the patient is sitting. The patient is moved forward in the chair, and he holds his hands clasped together, to avoid the temptation of pushing himself off his chair, or pulling onto the other chair, which would throw him off balance and increase his spasticity. The carer then holds him in the same way as if he was sitting on the side of the bed, with his head resting on her shoulder, and lifts him up and round onto the second chair. The *belt lift* is an alternative to the normal pelvic lift: the patient wears a strong webbing belt round the waist, and the carer pulls on this to lever the patient into position.

If the patient is very heavy, or the carer cannot manage for some other reason, the patient's moves during the day have to be carefully planned in advance, to ensure that two people can always be present. The pelvic lift can be done by two people. To lift the patient off the bed onto a chair or commode, one carer takes up the position already described, while the other stands behind the patient on the bed and guides the patient's seat up and round onto the chair. If the patient is being moved between two chairs, the second carer stands between the chairs, again behind the patient. In bed, the very heavy patient may be moved around with the *Australian lift*. Two people stand on either side of the bed, facing the patient. One brings the patient's head forward, so that he is sitting up but relaxed. His knees are bent. The carers then place one shoulder under the patient's shoulder nearest to them; they clasp their other hand to each other's wrist under the patient's thighs, balance on their free arms, and lever the patient upwards or downwards in the bed by bending their knees and leaning towards the direction of the movement.

A *transfer* involves guiding the patient in the correct movements to get up safely, and offering minimal help, in the situation where the patient can balance successfully. He may not have lost his ability to balance, or he may have relearned it through his therapy sessions. To get out of bed, the patient first lies on his back, clasps his hands together, keeping his elbows straight, and bends his unaffected knee, keeping his foot on the bed. The patient keeps his hands clasped together throughout the active parts of the transfer, so that he does not throw himself off balance by reaching out to grab the carer or the arm of the chair. He then turns onto his hemiplegic side when the carer tells him to, and the carer guides the movement with one hand on the patient's shoulder, the other on his pelvis. The carer lifts the patient's hemiplegic leg gently over the side of the bed, then places her hand on his stomach to stabilize him, and asks him to bring his other leg over beside the hemiplegic one. The carer puts one hand under the patient's head and round the back of his hemiplegic shoulder, presses down on his pelvis and guides the patient to sit up. With the patient sitting up with his feet flat on the floor, and the hemiplegic foot slightly forwards, the carer stands in front of the patient. The chair, wheelchair or commode onto which the patient is transferring is placed on one side of the carer, sideways on to the bed. The patient's hands are clasped together, with his arms straight, and the carer places her hands under his upper arms, to help bring his shoulders forwards. He then leans forward, and is guided up and round, so that he pivots to swing his hips round and onto the chair.

The patient's basic daily needs

Toileting

Going to the toilet is an important part of the day's activities, and is likely to be the first thing the patient does. The carer may find it repugnant at first to think of helping the patient with this basic human function. It may seem easier if you remember that all parents have to do just this when they change a baby's nappies, wipe the baby's bottom, and ensure it is clean and dry. At any age, good toilet hygiene is essential for preventing infections. For the hemiplegic patient, it requires extra care, because the patient is likely to be sitting still for much of the day, which in itself may make him more prone to infections, and the risk is magnified if there is any damp or dirty material next to his skin.

If the patient can stand and balance, he may be able to use the normal toilet. If he needs lifting, he is likely to need a commode, unless there is enough room around the toilet to allow for him to be lifted from a wheelchair to the toilet seat. The occupational therapist may supply portable handrails in the early stages after the stroke, so that the patient has some support on each side while he sits on the toilet, although these should not be used to lean on when standing up or sitting down. If the toilet seat is fairly low, the handrails may be fitted with a raised toilet seat between them, to fit over the toilet bowl, so that the patient can sit and stand more easily. Later on, permanent handrails may be fixed to the walls of the toilet, if necessary.

If the patient is safe sitting up, he should be left alone for privacy while he is passing urine or faeces, and he should have a bell to summon help, or perhaps a stick with which to knock on the wall or floor. The carer must ensure that the patient is cleaned thoroughly when he has finished. Non-allergenic, non-perfumed wet wipes (or baby wipes) are best for cleaning the anal area, to avoid the risk of faeces remaining clogged in the pubic hairs. After cleaning, the area should be dried most carefully with absorbent toilet paper or tissues. You should encourage the patient to clean himself while you guide him. If he cannot stand, the patient might be transferred to his bed before being cleaned, but if he is using a commode, it is usually possible to clean him from under the commode seat, once the pan of the commode has been taken out of the way.

Some hemiplegic patients are incontinent, either because they have poor sensation and cannot feel when the bladder or bowel needs to be emptied, or because they do not pay attention and so forget to go to the toilet, or ask to be taken. Toileting is a reflex, so they have to be taught control through a programme of toilet training. The patient is placed on the toilet or commode every two or three hours, and the carer carefully explains why each time. Inevitably, the incontinent patient needs cleaning and drying at very frequent intervals, to prevent infections such as cystitis. If the patient is usually in control of his bladder and bowels, but suddenly becomes incontinent, you should tell the doctor immediately, as it may be a sign of infection or problems.

Constipation can be a problem among hemiplegic patients, especially if they over-eat while they are doing less physical activity than normal. Changing the diet usually helps the constipation, especially if fibre is added. The doctor may refer the patient to a dietician for a specific regime, or he may prescribe a laxative to ease the congestion. The opposite problem of loose motions or diarrhoea should also be carefully monitored and corrected through altering the patient's diet.

If the patient needs to go to the toilet during the night, you should try to get him up. It may be more practical to use a commode for night-time toileting, even if the patient is capable of getting to the toilet when fully awake. Bottles and bed-pans are not really practical, partly because of the difficulty of positioning the patient properly to avoid increasing his spasticity, and partly because of the risk of unpleasant spillages.

Washing

If the patient was not admitted to hospital, or was discharged without having learned to wash himself properly, the community nurse attends to help him to wash, and to teach him and his carers how he can help himself. When she attends for the first time, she assesses the patient: if he is out of bed and eating his breakfast, for instance, she observes whether he can feed himself, or whether he needs help; whether he has perceptual problems; how good his balance is while he is sitting; whether he is limited by spasticity; what his posture is like; and then whether he is capable of standing and walking. The nurse also has to check the bathroom. There has to be enough space for her and the patient, and preferably room for the carer to watch the washing session as well. The floor should not be wet, polished or slippery, and there should not be loose rugs on it. If aids or alterations such as handrails or alarm buttons are likely to be needed, the nurse may liaise with the occupational therapist and social worker about having them supplied.

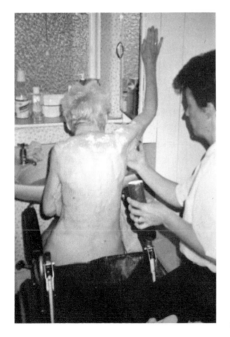

The patient holds the correct position during washing.

If he can, the patient walks into the bathroom with the nurse. If not, the nurse takes him in a wheelchair. If the wheelchair is too big to go into the bathroom, a Roamer chair may be supplied: this is a smaller chair on wheels, designed for short distances on flat surfaces. In the bathroom the nurse helps the patient to undress, taking care that he does not make any effort which increases his spasticity. She then teaches him to organize his toiletries and himself in the same way as she would in the hospital setting. The patient follows the same pattern of washing his face, then the rest of his body. The carer has to be involved in this process, so that every time the patient washes his face, hands or body, you help and remind him to do so correctly, without increasing his spasticity or putting himself into danger through careless movements. The message has to be reinforced all the time until the patient can wash himself properly and confidently, without losing concentration.

If the patient has good sitting balance, but not much standing balance, he may be able to sit in a hoist to be lifted into the bath. The hoist is rather like a ski-chair with a bar in front of the patient, and may be attached to the side of the bath. The patient remains sitting in it while washing, and is then lifted out. With good sitting balance, the patient can sit on a chair or stool in a shower compartment. This is a convenient way for the patient to wash himself all over, including his hair, provided there is room for the carer to help, if necessary. If the patient makes good progress physically, with good recovery of balance in sitting and then standing, he may be able to get into the bath. He might start by transferring himself from the wheelchair across onto a seat in the bath, and washing himself sitting up. A shower fitment on the bath taps facing the patient makes it easier for him to wash himself thoroughly. When he has good selective movements in his hemiplegic leg, he may be able to get down from the bath seat into the bath tub. A non-slip mat in the bottom of the bath may be needed for this. He needs excellent standing balance and selective leg movements to stand up and step into the bath, and even then he may need handrails on either side for stability and safety. He will not be allowed to try getting into the bath until he is capable of making all the necessary movements with full control, and no increase in his spasticity.

When you are helping the patient to wash, you should try to follow the same sequence as the nurse, and remember to keep describing to the patient everything that is happening. If he has severe perceptual problems, for instance, you may need to keep reminding him where his face is by helping him to touch it, or he may keep forgetting to shave or wash the left half of his face. The patient also has to learn to judge water temperature, and you have to be careful in the early stages that it is never too hot or cold for his comfort.

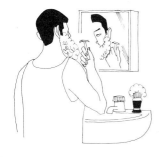

The patient with perceptual problems may need constant guidance when washing or shaving, to remind him that the affected half of his face exists.

Eating and drinking

Carers often find it difficult to cope with the problem of feeding the patient. Firstly, it involves a lot of work in terms of planning, preparation and serving the food. Secondly, hemiplegic patients often have difficulties eating, chewing and swallowing, and this can seem repulsive to the carer. If you do feel revolted when you watch the patient eat, you should not feel guilty about it, but neither should you let yourself become irritable with the patient over it. If he becomes nervous about eating, it will make his physical difficulties worse. The best thing is to discuss the situation with your doctor, social worker and family, and see if you can organize help for at least some of the meals.

If the patient cannot walk or be transported safely to the kitchen or the dining room, you have to bring the food to him. If this involves a fairly long distance through cold parts of the house, you may have to buy metal dish covers, plate warmers and Thermos flasks to keep the food and drinks warm. Food should not be too hot, however, so you should avoid serving piping hot boiled meals. You have to plan each meal to make sure both that the patient has a well balanced diet, and that you do not spend too much time and energy on journeys to and from the kitchen. For instance, it may help to keep salt, pepper and paper napkins in the bedroom, if that is where the patient eats his meals.

Eating is obviously a basic need, but it also forms part of the physical rehabilitation process. The patient has to be encouraged to eat his food correctly, as part of his recovery of control of his facial muscles. He must sit upright at a table to eat his meals: he cannot eat off a tray sitting in bed or an easy chair. Sitting in a good position for meals is an important part of the patient's recovery of sitting balance and control of his head movements. He should be able to sit close enough to the table to rest his hemiplegic arm comfortably on it. If his head tends to drop forward towards his plate as he eats, it may help to put the plate on a raised block on the table to reduce the distance from plate to face. To help his awareness of his affected side, you can arrange his place setting with the plate or bowl in front of him and his glass or cup in front of his hemiplegic side.

Eating a meal is a good time for socializing, so you should try to eat your own meal with the patient whenever possible, or organize family members or friends to do this. The patient may need help with eating. If he has a facial palsy, he may find it difficult to chew and swallow, and you can help this by encouraging him to chew and clear food from the hemiplegic side of his face. It can help if you gently stroke that side of his face as he eats: the physiotherapist will show you how to do this correctly. Especially at first, you may have to keep reminding the patient to sit upright and take the food to his mouth, rather than letting his face droop towards his plate. If he drools or loses food from the side of his mouth, you should help him to dab his mouth firmly with a folded napkin or handkerchief. (Wiping the mouth is discouraged, because it can over-stretch the delicate soft tissues and muscles.)

The choice of food you prepare depends partly on the patient's taste as to the food he prefers, partly on his eating abilities or difficulties, and partly on dietary needs such as avoiding putting on weight. If the patient can only use one hand, food should be prepared ready to eat, cut into manageable pieces. When preparing his food, you should think in terms of providing a 'finger buffet' with foods you might normally eat with a knife and fork. You may find the patient has little interest in food, so he may need encouraging to eat a little at a time. Overeating through boredom is a greater danger, so you should monitor the patient quite carefully to make sure he is not putting on excess weight. If you find it difficult to know how much, or what types of food the patient should eat, you can ask your doctor to refer the patient to a dietician.

For breakfast, suitable food might include toast in small squares or fingers (already spread with butter or jam or honey, if necessary), cereals in large chunks, and banana pieces. Bacon and bread can be eaten more easily as a sandwich than as separate items. The main meal of the day may be eaten at lunch time or in the evening, according to your normal habit. If the patient eats meat, it should be cut into chunks or cubes, not minced. A meat burger in a bun is easy to manage with one hand. Bones should be removed from chicken or fish. Salmon is relatively easy to eat, otherwise fish pie with pastry and leeks or fish cakes may be the best ways to eat fish. Vegetables should not be overcooked: firm *al dente* carrots, courgettes or cauliflower are easier to manage with a fork, and they help the patient to chew and swallow. Peas, sweetcorn and mushy soft vegetables, on the other hand, are likely to be too difficult to cope with. If the patient likes sauces on his food, it may be best to put a little directly on the relevant food. For dessert, pieces of fruit are generally the best option.

The patient may need to eat from a bowl at first, as he gets used to eating one-handed. A soup bowl with a flared rim can help prevent spillages. Similarly, a plate with a slight rim prevents food from sliding over the edge too easily. Some foods which are normally eaten on a plate, such as scrambled eggs, are best eaten from a cup or bowl and spooned up. The patient might manage to cut up his own food with a combined knife and fork, or he may even learn to cut his food with one hand, alternating cutting and eating using a normal knife and fork. Otherwise, chopsticks are practical for one-handed eating, if the food is cut up for the patient. Chopsticks have the added advantage that they prevent the patient from guzzling too much food in one mouthful. If the patient has problems holding his cutlery, he may need a thickened handle, usually made of rubber, which slides onto a knife, fork or spoon.

The patient should not be allowed to drink too much, as he would need to go to the toilet too often. Equally, he must drink enough to avoid dehydration. He should have a glass of water with each meal, at least, and possibly in between meals if his environment is very warm, or if he is doing a lot of active therapy. He may prefer still mineral water to tap water, so a bottle can be kept near him. Acid drinks like orange juice should not be taken in large quantities: it may be preferable to squeeze or liquidize fresh fruit and dilute it with plain water, if the patient particularly likes fruit juices. Tea and coffee should be strictly limited, and the patient should drink them from a small cup, and should not be given several cups in succession. Alcoholic drinks should only be given if the doctor allows it, and the patient must not be allowed to drink excessive amounts of alcohol.

The patient should be encouraged to drink from a cup or glass with both hands clasped round it. If he uses one hand on the cup handle, he should always have the other hemiplegic hand correctly positioned in front of him. It is better for the patient to use a shallow cup rather than a deeper mug, partly to prevent an excessive fluid intake, and partly because he may have difficulty in judging the depth of a mug and so may tend to spill his drink. A useful type of cup has a cut-out piece opposite the drinking side, so that the patient can tip the cup up against his face without hitting the bridge of his nose.

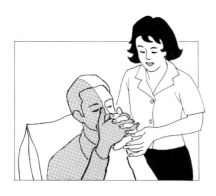

Drinking from a cup.

Dressing

The patient should not be expected to get dressed in the early stages following his stroke. If he cannot put his clothes on himself, learning to get dressed is a necessary part of his rehabilitation programme. Some patients relearn dressing very quickly, others extremely slowly. The patient should not be pressurized. Initially, it may be as much as he can manage to co-operate in changing his pyjamas, a relatively simple task with proper guidance. He may need to stay in pyjamas and dressing gown for a long time until he can learn how to cope with normal clothes. If you make him feel that he should be getting dressed, and he tries to do so before he is ready, in rehabilitation terms, he will certainly increase his spasticity and make himself even less capable of learning the movements. If you force his limbs into clothes, the same effect follows: in the arm this can cause severe shoulder pain which will hold up the patient's rehabilitation. The worst mistake is to leave clothes near the patient when he is unattended: he may fall over if he tries to put them on by himself, as he may not yet have realized that he cannot balance and move normally.

Getting dressed consists of a complex sequence of movements depending on the patient's ability to balance and co-ordinate his actions. Dressing is a two-handed activity which is extremely difficult to do with only one hand. It involves co-operation between both sides of the body: for instance, as one leg is put into a trouser-leg, the other holds the body upright; a sweater has to be pulled over the head and then organized so that one's arms can slide into the sleeves. Buttons and zips are difficult to manipulate without one hand holding the garment steady. Apart from the difficulties of physically getting into clothes and fastening them, the patient also has to identify what each garment is, which way it goes on, and to which part of the body each part of each garment belongs. For the patient with figure-ground perceptual problems this selection and identification process is virtually impossible. He has to relearn it stage by stage, building up his awareness through experience, in much the same way as a child learns about putting on clothes by himself.

If the patient *has* to get dressed before he is able to dress independently, you have to dress him with care, so that he does not get involved in making any effort. The carer learns how to dress the patient in the right way from the occupational therapist or physiotherapist. All the clothes are chosen carefully, so that you can get them on without discomfort to the patient. Sometimes, in hospital, patients are not given underwear, even when they wear outer clothes, so that toileting is easier. However, this often makes the patient feel vulnerable. It is probably preferable for the patient to have underwear if at all possible, for normal dignity. While you are dressing him, you should make the patient aware of what you are doing by naming each garment as you put it on, and showing him that it is the right way round. Although he must not make any physical effort, you should allow him to follow the sequence of movements that you are making, and tell him what you are doing and why. Repeating the verbal descriptions is specially important for the patient with perceptual and speech difficulties, as it helps him to become familiar with the planning needed for each item of clothing.

The stage at which the patient starts relearning how to dress himself is determined largely by his progress in regaining his balance firstly while sitting up and then standing. Good co-operation between the physiotherapist, occupational therapist and nurse is vital: the patient must not be taught several different ways of doing the same dressing task, nor must he be given tasks which he cannot achieve. Everyone involved has to realize that the tasks are not relearned in an automatic sequence: the fact that the patient may be able to put on his sweater one day does not necessarily mean that he is immediately able to progress to putting on his trousers – indeed, he may have forgotten how to cope with the sweater the following day.

The therapist assesses what the patient should start with: he automatically starts with a pyjama jacket, if he has difficulties with this. He then progresses to a simple upper body garment, such as a sleeveless vest or loose T-shirt. Getting into a shirt comes at a later stage, a sweater later still. Shoes and socks are tackled before trousers, and track-suit trousers with an elasticated waist would be chosen for either a male or a female patient. Underpants and knickers are harder to manage, so they are practised at a later stage.

All clothing is chosen in slightly larger sizes than normal, so that it is not too tight, and it is easier to slip on. Fastenings are made as simple as possible: ladies might use an all-in-one slip-over brassière, or one with front fastening; shoes might have velcro or elastic laces rather than normal laces; shirts would use velcro strips rather than buttons; men's trousers would have a zip fly rather than buttons, with a velcro fastening at the top; braces are easier to manage than a belt to hold trousers up; a lady's skirt might have an elasticated waist or a velcro fastening. For a very large female patient, or one who has extremely poor balance, a wrap-around skirt may be more practical. A normal, loose-fitting skirt can be split up the side and fitting with a Velcro fastening. This makes it very easy to put on and take off, even when the patient is sitting down.

When dressing practice starts, the patient is carefully positioned so that his hemiplegic arm and leg are well supported. He has to be able to sit upright in his chair using his trunk muscles, without pulling or pushing himself up using his unaffected arm. He may sit at a table, which has to be big enough to spread the garment out on it. If the garment is a shirt, the front faces the patient. The hemiplegic arm rests on the garment: if the therapist lifts it, she takes the shoulder and hand. The patient is taught to lift his arm by gripping it behind the elbow with his other hand, drawing it gently forwards and up keeping the elbow straight, palm facing upwards, as he leans forwards from the hips. The sleeve for the hemiplegic arm is gathered together, and the unaffected hand goes into it from the cuff, in order to draw the hemiplegic hand into the sleeve up to the wrist. The sleeve is straightened out up the arm with gentle stroking movements by the unaffected hand. To hold the sleeve up, the patient may take the collar between his teeth while he reaches behind his neck to bring the shirt behind his back. Alternatively, he might spread the front of the shirt across his body to stop it from slipping down his arm. Leaning forwards, the patient then slides his unaffected arm into the second sleeve. He sits up straight to do up the buttons or velcro fastenings. The only fastening he cannot reach is the cuff on the unaffected arm.

A sweater is placed with the back uppermost, and the hemiplegic arm is placed beside the sweater. The sleeve is drawn up, put over the hemiplegic arm, and drawn gently upwards. The patient pulls the sweater over his head and then puts the unaffected arm into its sleeve. Alternatively, the unaffected arm is put into its sleeve and the patient then pulls the sweater over his head, leaning well forwards from the hips. The latter method requires very good balance in sitting, together with good forward mobility.

For trousers, socks and shoes, the garments are placed on a stool slightly to the side of the patient. The shoes and socks might be on the floor if the patient is capable of reaching down for them. The garments might be placed by his hemiplegic side, if there is no risk of him falling as he reaches for them, and if he is beginning to use the hemiplegic arm. To put the trousers, socks and shoes on, the patient sits in a chair, and lifts his hemiplegic leg to cross over the other leg. If he cannot lift the leg unaided, he may move it by clasping his hands together just below the knee, holding the shin bone firmly, and using his hands to lift the leg up, shifting his weight sideways towards his unaffected side as he does so. Another method is to grip under the lower calf with the unaffected hand to lift the hemiplegic leg across. If the patient cannot lift the leg across, the therapist helps by supporting it under the foot and thigh, and taking it up gently. The patient puts the sock on his hemiplegic foot, then pulls the trouser leg on up over the knee, and then puts the shoe on the foot. (The sock is usually prepared by the therapist, who rolls the top over.) The hemiplegic leg is then lifted back to the floor, the trouser leg is pulled a little further up the thigh, and anchored in place by the patient crossing his unaffected leg over it. The patient puts the sock on his unaffected foot. He holds the trouser tightly outwards as he puts the unaffected leg into it, crosses this leg over the other again, and puts his shoe on. He stands up with the assistance of the therapist: he may do his trousers up while the therapist makes sure he remains properly aligned and upright, or the therapist may fasten the trousers while the patient concentrates on standing and balancing.

Undressing is easier than dressing, as it does not involve so much planning, so even the patient with perceptual problems can generally manage. It is generally done as a reverse of the sequence for dressing. The patient often learns to undress by himself long before he can manage to dress. The therapist may encourage him to practise taking off clothes by himself, having helped him to put them on, to build up his awareness and confidence. The patient has to undress slowly and methodically, as there is a temptation to go too quickly, which might make him lose his balance and increase his spasticity. For ease, upper garments like a sweater or shirt are pulled over the head first, and the hemiplegic arm comes out of its sleeve last. Trousers are unfastened with the patient sitting down, dropped with the patient standing, and then removed with the patient sitting down. The trouser, sock and shoe come off the hemiplegic leg last.

No patient is expected to learn all the parts of these sequences in one go. Some of the movements may be modified according to the patient's abilities and limitations. The process usually starts with practice of the initial movements for putting on a particular garment, before the garment is given to the patient. The first sessions may be limited to the patient learning how to move his body, arm or leg into the right positions, while the therapist performs most of the actual dressing. The carer is involved in the routine: you will watch the therapist at first, and then learn how much you can do to help the learning process at any stage. The therapist will show you the techniques of helping the patient to cope with particular garments. Gradually, as the patient learns how to dress himself, at least in part, the movement patterns become part of normal everyday life, and dressing becomes part of the patient's increasingly independent activities.

Activities, social life and work

The patient should not stay in bed without a special reason, such as feeling ill or exceptionally fatigued, or having a headache. Even then, if at all possible, he should get up for meals. He must not be allowed to think that staying in bed would solve the physical problems of his hemiplegia, as the opposite would certainly happen: he would become lazy, weak, and his spasticity would become more entrenched and pronounced. It is usually a waste of time trying to explain the dangers, especially if the patient feels in a self-pitying mood. Nor is it helpful to argue or get angry about it. You simply have to try to organize each day so that the patient has enough, but not too many, useful, interesting and pleasurable activities to occupy him.

The choice of suitable activities is best made in consultation with the physiotherapist, occupational therapist and speech therapist, as they will be able to suggest the most appropriate pastimes to help the patient's mental and physical needs. There may be appointments to keep, perhaps for treatment sessions with the physiotherapist or speech therapist. These engagements and meal times should be considered the fixed points in each day. Other activities are planned around them. To programme the day successfully, you need to take into account how tired the patient is likely to be, for instance after a physiotherapy treatment session. If he has a tiring morning session, for instance, he may need a rest period in his chair or in bed after lunch. After the rest he should be involved in some activitiy which does not require too much physical effort. As he gets fitter, he may be able to do two or three physically demanding sessions each day, interspersed with lighter activities and rest periods. Whatever he is doing, you must remember that he must be positioned correctly at all times to prevent his spasticity from increasing.

While physical fatigue is one problem which needs careful control, boredom and lack of motivation are potentially far more difficult to combat. It takes a great deal of sensitivity to provide activities which stimulate the patient's interest, without exhausting him or making him frustrated if he cannot achieve what he wants or what you hope for. You need to

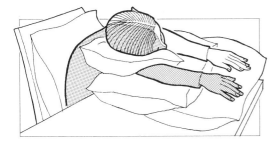

The patient resting, sitting in the chair.

encourage the patient with gentleness, but you will probably have to be firm if he wants to stop a task simply because he feels bored and lazy. While you can substitute another activity for one the patient wants to abandon, you should not allow him to stop and do nothing. The more time in the day the patient is idle, the more he is likely to sink into a torpor of laziness. It is specially important not to let him vegetate in front of the television for long periods. If possible, he should not have a television in the room where he spends most of his time. If he does, it should certainly not be on all the time. Television watching should be selective, and you should try to discuss the programmes watched with the patient, or relate them to pictures and stories in books or magazines, so that some intellectual stimulus is involved.

Activities in the home

Having consulted the therapists about the best type of activity to choose for the patient, you may be able to work out how best to interest and amuse the patient through your knowledge of what he enjoyed doing before his stroke or head injury.

If the patient has perceptual problems, it is useful to draw or tape a line down the centre of his personal table, to help him differentiate between left and right. Using a fluorescent marker to highlight the left side of any reading material, such as a newspaper, can help the patient to pay attention to the whole text instead of just the right half. Jigsaws with large pieces help the patient to relearn how to match up shapes and images. You may have to help him at first, but as he progresses, he can tackle more complicated puzzles. Many of the toys suitable for teaching very young children about matching objects, shapes and colours can help the patient with severe perceptual difficulties. Games like dominoes and draughts can help both perception and memory. The patient may find these actvities both boring and frustrating, especially if you are constantly trying to make him concentrate on them as educational tasks. Children in the family, such as grandchildren, nephews or nieces, can help by sharing these activities with the patient. They are more likely to enjoy the games themselves, and so can help the patient to have fun as he goes through the relearning process.

The patient's memory can be retrained through simple exercises such as question-and-answer sessions after you have read him a short passage from a book or newspaper. Radio programmes or 'talking book' tape recordings can be used for the same purpose. Reading and listening can also help with speech and comprehension problems. You can make up simple, large crossword puzzles for the patient to solve. He can practise forming as many words as possible from one long word or a collection of single letters: the letter units from a Scrabble set are useful for this purpose. The patient with mild speech and comprehension problems may enjoy playing Scrabble itself. He may even be able to tackle learning a foreign language. On the other hand, for a patient with severe word-finding difficulties, you may have to label all the normal objects round the home, and ask the patient to say the name of the object and point to it every time he wants something.

Learning handwriting with the non-dominant hand is difficult, so it usually comes at a late stage of recovery. However, it is useful for the patient to practise writing words, so a typewriter or word-processor can be the answer. It is slightly easier to feed paper one-handed into a word-processor than a typewriter. A manual typewriter is physically harder to use than an electric keyboard. If the patient is at the stage where he can write business or personal letters, he will probably prefer to use a modern electric machine or word-processor so that he can correct any errors easily and neatly.

If the patient had hobbies before his stroke or head injury, such as drawing, painting or needlepoint, you should try to make it possible for him to take them up again. It is usually easy to secure a canvas or needlepoint frame in clamps so that the patient can work one-handed on them. If he does not enjoy his previous hobbies because he cannot achieve his former standards, you can try introducing him to new, different ones. It sometimes helps if you choose something you have not done before either, but which interests you, so that you can share the activity on equal terms.

Conversation is an important part of reviving the patient's ability to communicate and his interest in the world around him. Your direct communication with the patient is a vital part of your care, so you should try to keep a time spare for simple conversation, no matter how busy you are with organizing the practical aspects of home life and the patient's needs. Visiting friends can be a great help for this, and you can ask them to come prepared with items to read to the patient, or ideas to discuss. The patient may also like talking to friends on the telephone. If he cannot look up names and numbers in his address book, he may be able to memorize the order of a list of people whose numbers are entered into the memory of a modern telephone. Then all he has to do is to press one digit, and the number is automatically dialled for him.

Working in the kitchen is a more practical way for the patient to relearn relevant skills. He may need special implements, such as a wall-mounted tin opener which he can operate with one hand. Your occupational therapist or physiotherapist will advise you about the many ingenious gadgets available which might be useful. The patient may be able to wash up or cook, and practise planning and problem-solving. Cooking from a recipe is a good exercise in reading, comprehension and translation of concepts into actions. Even looking around the kitchen in order to make up the shopping lists is a task involving observation, forward thinking and memory.

Some activities in the kitchen can be done sitting in a wheelchair. However, once the patient can stand and balance successfully, he can stand at the sink, and perhaps move sideways using the kitchen units for support, so the exercise also involves the physical work of balancing and transferring weight. You may need to stand behind the patient at first, to encourage him to move correctly and not in a 'dot and carry' pattern. You may also need to supervise the patient, in case he forgets what he has to do and leaves the gas on without lighting it, for example, or without putting the pan of food on the cooker. He may get muddled, and perhaps put dirty clothes into the oven instead of the washing machine, or food into the dustbin instead of the saucepan. You may need to keep repeating the names of foods and objects to reinforce his awareness, or to recite the order in which a task like cooking or washing up is achieved.

Gardening

The patient may have enjoyed gardening before his stroke or head injury, and it is an activity he can return to even with quite a degree of disability. If he took no interest in gardening before his illness, he may find it refreshing to be outdoors looking at the different colours and shapes of the plants, smelling their fragrance, and watching the insects and birds they attract. If it is warm enough for the patient to sit in the garden, he may enjoy just watching all the garden life. However, he is likely to feel much more satisfied if he can take an active part in looking after the plants. The garden can provide the patient's first opportunity to feel he has achieved something by himself: he can grow flowers to beautify the garden or provide cut flowers for the house, or he might grow vegetables or herbs.

You will have to work out the potential problems for the patient, and take care to avoid them. You may have to organize the access to the garden for the patient. If there are steps, he may need handrails if he is walking, or a ramp if he moves about in a wheelchair. Wide paths are needed for a wheelchair, and the paths need to be smooth and free of weeds. If the patient is walking, you have to be careful that the path is not slippery at all when he first goes outside. It may need hosing at high pressure to get rid of any surface slime. There may be areas of the garden which are specially suitable for the patient to work in: he needs to be able to reach the soil with his hands or tools without risking scratching himself on thorny plants or hitting his head or eyes on jutting or overhanging branches. Canes which support tall plants should have a cover over the exposed end, so that they are clearly visible and do not risk poking the patient in the eye when he bends over, or if he slips. A soft rubber ball like a squash ball is easy to insert over each cane: your local squash club may be willing to give you discarded punctured balls.

The patient may not have full feeling in the skin on his hemiplegic side, so he should cover his arms and legs with clothing and both his hands with gardening gloves, unless it is really too hot for comfort. If the weather is very sunny, the patient should wear a sun-hat and neckerchief, and he must drink water at frequent intervals. You may need to watch him at first, so that you can clean and dress any grazes or cuts immediately. Like any other gardener, the patient should be protected by anti-tetanus inoculations, so you should check with your doctor to make sure these are kept up to date.

Raised flower beds are ideal for people in wheelchairs. Some flower beds may have soft, fertile soil which is easier to dig or hoe than hard or stony ground. The patient who can stand and balance can work standing up, so he can probably tackle every job in the garden, from digging and weeding to mowing the lawn. However, he is likely to need to rest at frequent intervals. A small seat, which also serves as a kneeler when it is turned upside down, is a practical item which can be carried in one hand. If there are comfortable and solid garden chairs around the garden, the patient can rest and relax in them when he needs to.

If the patient has recovered the use of his affected hand, he may be able to do jobs like digging and trimming the lawn. He should work with lightweight tools: his spade, for example, should have a small blade. Tools with extra long handles save him from having to bend over too far, which might undermine his balance. If the affected arm is still disabled, the patient may still manage to link both hands round the handles of tools such as a hoe, rake or spade. Otherwise he is restricted to those jobs which he can do one-handed. Many garden tools are adapted for disabled people. You can get every variety of fork, weeder, hoe, trowel or rake with long, medium or short handles. Some implements are set with the heads at different angles to make them easier to manoeuvre with one hand.

The patient may need help with organizing the tools and trying out new tasks at first. If you have a shed, the tools need to be neatly arranged, each in its proper place. A gardener's belt, with clasps and pouches for small tools is a practical way of carrying the tools around. For larger items, a holdall like a sports bag can be useful. If every tool is replaced in the belt or holdall after use, you will have less of a problem with tools being forgotten and left in odd corners. All tools should then be returned to the shed or storage place where they are easily accessible.

Each session in the garden should be planned, so that the patient has a specific aim, such as weeding or planting flowers in a certain patch. If he is an experienced gardener, you have to make sure that he sets himself achievable targets, and does not become over-ambitious. If he has not done much gardening before, you can work together, so that you can enjoy sharing the tasks, and it is easier for you to assess when the patient has had enough.

If you do not have a garden, or if the access to your garden is too difficult for the patient, he can still enjoy doing smaller-scale gardening work using planters, tubs or pots. These may be on a window-sill, balcony or patio, and are often more convenient to manage because there is a firm, hard surface to stand on, or to take the wheelchair. The soil level is raised, so the patient can reach it without having to bend too far. The patient may have to move about in a relatively confined area, so you have to make sure he can do so safely before he begins.

Apart from enjoying the achievement of working on his own garden, the patient may also like to visit parks and gardens open to the public. Most should allow for wheelchair access, but you should always check by reading any brochures or information sheets, or telephoning before you go. There may also be local gardening clubs or allotment societies which the patient can join in order to meet other gardeners, disabled or able-bodied. The benefits of gardening as a hobby are wide-ranging: it is satisfying as a pastime with a visible end-product, and it offers a lot of opportunities for meeting like-minded people in a pleasant environment. If you want to find out more about gardening for the disabled before the patient starts, you can ask your occupational therapist for advice and available literature, look up books on the subject in your local library, or contact specialist organizations such as The Garden Club, the Gardens for the Disabled Trust, or the Royal Horticultural Society.

Sports

Many stroke and head-injured patients return to sports when they feel well enough. They may even take up new sports which they had never tried before. Many sports can be played and enjoyed one-handed, even if this does limit the player's performance a little. Walking, cycling and swimming are healthy exercise which can help keep the patient's blood pressure down, if he does them sensibly, without putting himself under undue pressure. Sports like bowls and snooker are excellent practice for standing balance, if the patient has recovered good balance and selective movements in his leg. Equally, there are many games which can be played from a wheelchair, if the patient cannot stand, but his sitting balance is good. There are many opportunities for disabled people to join in team or individual sports, and within some sports people with handicaps can participate with able-bodied people. Two organizations which advise on sports for the disabled are the British Sports Association for the Disabled, and 'Les Autres Sports'.

If he wants to take up sports again, the patient must be guided by his physiotherapist, so that he does not attempt exercises which are too hard, which would inevitably increase his spasticity. His sports activities have to be carefully chosen and graded. He should be encouraged to think of sport as healthy exercise done for fun, rather than for competition. If he was involved in competitive sports before, aiming from the start at tournaments and championships places a lot of pressure on the patient, and it may lead to bitter frustration when he cannot reach his previous standards as quickly as he might hope. Returning to competitions should be a long-term aim, provided the physiotherapist and the carers feel it is realistic.

It is important for the patient to be aware of the limitations

likely to be caused by his spasticity. If he does sport independently, he has to concentrate on maintaining control over
any associated reactions which could knock him off balance
as he makes a physical effort. If he has sports coaching or
attends exercise classes where the instructor is not aware of
the particular problems of spasticity, he should take care not
to try any movement he is not capable of. It is also true that
exercise classes arranged specifically for hemiplegic patients
are sometimes organized by people who are not aware of
the nature of spasticity, so the carer and the patient must
scrutinize any proposed activities before the patient tries to
join in.

Going out with the carer

The patient should get out of the house at intervals, if at all
possible. If the access to your front door is difficult, perhaps
with steps, you may need to have a ramp made, if the patient
is still in a wheelchair. If the patient cannot walk at all, you
should have a special wheelchair for outdoor use; while an
indoor wheelchair has large back wheels and relatively thin
tyres, the outdoor version may have four small wheels with
thick fat tyres, which should be kept pumped up to the
correct pressure. If the patient can walk, but your steps
have no handrails, you should try to have secure rails fitted,
preferably on both sides of the steps. The social services and
your community occupational therapist can advise and help
you in this. Otherwise, it may be easier for the patient to
come out of the back door and walk or be wheeled out
through a side gate, if it is all on a level.

For the first few trips outside, you should plan only to go
a short way, so that the patient can get used to the distracting
sights and sounds. Even if he is walking well, you may need
to take a wheelchair in case he gets tired, or you can plan the
outing so that you walk short distances between benches in
the street or local park. If you do take a wheelchair out with
you, never forget the support cushion for the seat, and make
sure the footplates are always in place. The patient should
sit correctly at all times: he should not have to hold his
hemiplegic leg up with his unaffected leg, as this is tiring for
him, and creates the danger that his outstretched legs might

easily be jarred or hit. You should teach the patient safety measures when going outside with the wheelchair: for instance, he must keep his hemiplegic arm safely on his lap, and he must always check that both feet are on the footplates before you set off. You should always double-check that the patient is sitting up safely, and keep watch in case he changes position as you go along. When you push the chair down kerbs or ramps it is safest to go down backwards, as the patient might fall out of the chair if he is facing forwards as the chair tilts downwards.

The patient may also need to practise being a passenger in the car: getting in and out may be difficult, so you may need help from the occupational therapist or physiotherapist to find the easiest way of managing. Some cars can be fitted with a passenger seat which swings outwards at the touch of a lever to face the door, so that the patient does not have to twist to enter or leave the car. If the patient still needs to use a wheelchair, you will need one which is fully portable and the right size to fit into the back of the car. When you lift the wheelchair into the car, you should fold it so that it is sideways in front of you, with the handles to one side and clipped up; then lean over the chair to grasp the cross-bar under the seat; lift the chair up, step back with one leg, lever the wheelchair towards you, over your thighs, and then slide it into the boot, wheels first.

If your car seems totally unsuitable for transporting the patient, you may have to exchange it for a different model. A three-door hatchback car may be more practical for the patient, because the front doors tend to be slightly bigger than in four-door cars, and there is plenty of room for the wheelchair in the back. An estate car provides even more luggage space. If the car is low to the ground, it is likely to be extremely difficult for the patient to get in and out, so you might try using a car in which you can raise and lower the suspension. If you are taking the patient out frequently, and rely on the car as his necessary transport, you should qualify for a disabled permit to park in restricted areas. You may also qualify for a Mobility Allowance to help pay transport costs such as the Road Tax, or other grants such as an interest-free loan towards the purchase of a new car. Your social worker should be able to advise you about these.

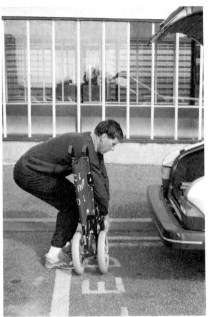 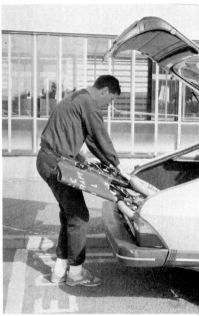

Lifting the wheelchair into the car: bend your knees to lift the wheelchair up, then slide it into the car boot.

Once the patient is used to getting out of the house, he can go out for social occasions. These may be organized by local groups such as stroke clubs, so that patients and their carers get together for outings or entertainments and shows. However, the patient may also like to go out to the cinema, theatre, concert hall, pub or restaurant in the normal way. Facilities for wheelchairs in public places are variable in Britain. The Disability Information Service Surrey (DISS) holds computerized information on facilities for disabled people throughout Britain. You should telephone before venturing to a place for the first time, but it is probably wise also to go by yourself and have a look, to check whether you can manoeuvre the patient in and out of the building easily, and whether the toilet facilities are suitable. If the patient can walk, you should make sure the access into the building is not too difficult.

If you go to a restaurant, it is worth telephoning beforehand to inform the staff that you are coming with a disabled person, so that you can reserve a table at a convenient distance from the front door or the toilet. If the restaurant has flimsy chairs or hard benches, you can ask for an upright chair with cushions and arms to be provided, so that the patient can sit in the correct position. You can also ask for the patient's meal to be cut up in the kitchen ready to eat, although this is something that can be done when you order the meal. The patient may feel embarrassed at first when he goes to places he does not know, but he will be made welcome if the restaurateur knows what to expect. A few successful trips to restaurants will not only be enjoyable for the patient, but they will boost his confidence and help him to realize that he can take part in normal social life.

Going out independently

When the patient can walk safely, he may wish to go out alone, and you should encourage him to do this. In order to be safe outside, the patient must be aware of his limitations. Therefore, it is a good idea to 'practise' going out, so that the patient can find out how he copes. You can plan the first outing as a short walk down the road and back: the patient walks ahead, while you follow at some distance, in case he gets into difficulties. There are some predictable problems which might arise when the patient first goes out alone. He may tend to walk slightly sideways towards his hemiplegic side, and therefore bump into people or objects, which can be embarrassing. He is likely to be easily distracted by the sights and sounds around him, and this might make him stray into the road or trip and fall. He may go too far for his capabilities and get too tired to walk back safely. He may be frightened by crossing a road, by fast cars, by crowds or sudden noises, so that his spasticity increases; he may panic and freeze in these situations, so that he cannot move at all. The patient has to experience walking outside in order to overcome these problems, so he might do several 'practice walks' before venturing out without you following. It may help him to take his wheelchair out at first: pushing it may help him to balance more easily. The wheelchair provides the ideal type of support, as the patient cannot lean on it as he would on a walking frame, because the chair would tip up. It may also be useful in case the patient becomes unexpectedly tired, and needs to sit down for a moment.

When he is walking outside, the patient has to be specially careful to lift his feet off the ground so that he does not trip. He also has to learn not to watch his feet, because bending his head downwards will probably increase his spasticity, and make him more likely to fall. Looking down carries the further risk of making him unaware of other dangers around him. When he can walk outside confidently, the patient can plan to increase the distance he walks, or to go on the same route, but taking less time to complete his walk. This type of training helps the patient to walk further without losing his ability to walk correctly. Crossing roads is always frightening at first, and the patient may have to relearn how to use pelican and zebra crossings. If he feels very unsafe, because the traffic is moving fast, he may prefer to ask a passer-by to help him across the road. If he does, he should ask the helper simply to make sure that the cars stop for long enough to allow him to cross: the helper should not take the patient's arm and hurry him across. If the patient cannot speak well enough to explain all this, he can carry a card explaining his problem, and what kind of help he needs. Motorists should always remember that someone who is having difficulty crossing a road quickly may be panic-stricken by revving engines or impatient horn-sounding. This is especially true for older people. Drivers and riders should always stop still at pedestrian crossings, and not pull forwards until the person is safely on the pavement.

The patient with perceptual problems who cannot judge distances should not be allowed to go out alone into situations where he will have to cross roads. In order to help the patient learn to judge distances, you can practise crossing roads with him, pointing out how far away any oncoming traffic is, and telling the patient whether there is time to cross the road, and, if so, how much time you have to get across. Some patients, especially after a head injury, may become disorientated while they are out, so that they cannot find their way home. If this is likely to happen, the patient should certainly wear a 'dog-tag' or carry an identity card with his name and address on it. He might also wear an electronic tag on his wrist, so that the carer can always pinpoint where he is.

When the patient is out alone, he may need to use taxis or public transport to get around. He has to practise using buses and trains, perhaps going first with the carer, then with the carer following, and finally on his own. Taxis are obviously easier to use, but if the patient cannot speak properly, he may need to use clearly written cards to explain to the taxi driver why he cannot speak, and where he wants to go. Even if the patient cannot read properly, he may, with practice, be able to identify the appropriate card in a card index system, if the cards are very clearly presented, and perhaps colour coded as well. Planning each outing is good training for the patient: if he has difficulties with programming, you might go over the plan with him each time before he goes out, and ask him to say out loud exactly where he is going and how he is going to get there.

For greater mobility, the patient might learn to ride a tricycle or a bicycle with stabilizers, so that he can travel further and carry loads. A motorized scooter or buggy provides more mobility with less effort. In all cases, the patient should learn how to control the vehicle with absolute confidence before venturing out in it, and he must obey the rules for road safety. If the general practitioner pronounces the patient fit enough, he may be able to start driving a car again, although he may need to retake a driving test if he has not been able to drive for several months. His car may need to be specially adapted, for instance if he cannot use his hemiplegic hand to operate controls or the hand brake. The Banstead Place Mobility Centre has full facilities for training disabled drivers and for assessing what alterations their vehicles might need. When the patient restarts driving, he may gain confidence by having lessons through one of the major driving schools, such as the British School of Motoring (BSM), which have specialist intructors for people with physical handicaps who are learning or relearning driving. He can ask the school, the major motoring associations, his social worker or his general practitioner whether he needs to attend one of the recognized centres for handicapped drivers. In any case, he has to notify the Drivers' Medical Branch of the Driver and Vehicle Licensing Centre if he has any kind of disability when he resumes driving. On no account should he be allowed simply to get in his car and drive around before he has been pronounced competent to drive, and has organized his driving licence and insurance accordingly, if for no other reason than that his insurance would be invalid if he did have an accident.

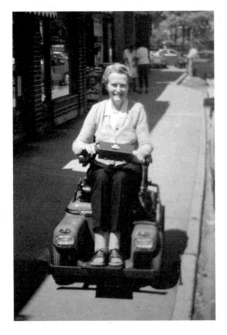

A motorized buggy provides independent mobility.

If the patient cannot walk, he may still be able to go out independently in a wheelchair. For short outings, he may be able to operate an ordinary wheelchair, but driving these one-handed requires enormous effort, so an electrically operated wheelchair is preferable. This at least gives him the freedom to go out for air and to do errands such as visiting local shops or going to the hairdresser. It also gives him practice in planning outings and taking some responsibility for his own actions. If relearning to walk safely takes several months, going out in a wheelchair alone can prevent the patient from feeling too housebound and frustratingly dependent on other people for his mobility.

Going back to work

In Britain most people who are in full-time contracted employment receive full pay for six months, followed by half pay for a further six months, if they have a serious illness or accident which prevents them from working. In the early stages of recovery following a stroke or head injury, it may seem impossible that the patient will ever be able to work again. If the patient is already close to retirement age, and prefers to take early retirement if sufficient benefits are available, then it may be sensible to take this option. However, if the patient is younger, and would wish to return to work, you should not make any hasty decisions about the patient's long-term prospects of returning to employment. Remember that recovery is a slow but continuing process, and that there is no doubt that the patient will improve, provided he does not have any major setbacks.

The patient who was self-employed with his own business before his illness may have much greater financial difficulties than the employed worker. He may also face the prospect of long-term hardship, if he cannot return to work at all. This is one of the reasons why anyone who works for himself should make sure that he is fully covered by insurance providing for loss of earnings during a long-term illness, as well as insurance against the possibility that he might not be able to work again after such an illness. If money is short while the patient is ill, there is great pressure on the carer and the family, and often it may mean that the patient is unable to receive the specialist rehabilitation treatment which is increasingly difficult to obtain under the National Health Service. If poverty is a long-term prospect, it is likely also to affect the morale of the patient and his carers.

However, the patient may be able to return to his own job, when he is sufficiently recovered. On the other hand, he may no longer be capable of doing what he did before, although he could still cope with other kinds of work. A welder, for instance, may not recover sufficient balance or hand control to go back to welding, but he may be able to work light machinery. In many cases companies might find alternative work for their employees, or even create new jobs for them within their capabilities. British companies are beginning to be more aware of the needs of their disabled employees, and the potential benefits of continuing their employment. However, it has to be said that the British lag behind other European countries, particularly Germany, in this respect.

If the patient has problems with his employer, he may need to apply for professional help through his social worker. The Disablement Resettlement Officer, a government official, has the brief of settling disabled people into full, useful employment. If he cannot persuade a former employer to take the patient back, he may be able to find suitable alternative work through his knowledge of other companies. He can often find suitable work for the previously self-employed patient. For the young patient with a stroke or head injury, work may be found in specialized government sheltered workshops, where disabled workers have facilities and staff tailored for them. The largest company employing disabled people in Britain is Remploy, which is run as a profit-making business, but equipped with machinery specially made for use by the disabled, and supervisors who are trained to help the disabled staff cope.

When the patient returns to work, he will probably have to work part-time at first, as he gets used to the discipline and pressures of working again. A woman who has recovered from a stroke or head injury may decide she would like to work for the first time, as part of the challenge of overcoming her illness. She too should find suitable work, and start with just a few hours, perhaps one or two days a week, before building up towards full-time work if she wishes. The carer should always be positive if the patient does have the ability and opportunity to return to work. It may involve you in extra duties and worries at first: for instance, you may have to take the patient to his workplace by car, and collect him again, and the timing may not be convenient for you. You may have to organize different kinds of help in the home, if the patient has been doing tasks and housework. You may worry if the patient gets very tired or anxious about his situation. You may need to help the patient at work, especially if he is returning to his own business. However, if you and he can overcome the early period and settle back into regular work routines, it is a vital part of his full recovery.

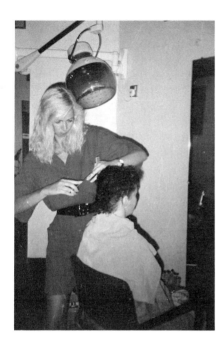

Back to work hairdressing after a stroke: standing all day and using both hands with precision.

Caring for the carer

In the early stages of recovery following a stroke or head injury, you, as carer, have to be nurse, therapist, friend and companion to the patient. It can be an isolating experience. The patient's condition might change only slowly, as he can go on recovering over several years. Your ultimate aim is to help the patient back towards normal life, if possible, so you should try to help him keep in touch with friends and acquaintances. This is another reason for you to maintain your own social life, or to build up a new network of friends, if necessary. If you have a wide range of social activities, the patient may be able to join in some of them with you, even if he cannot resume his former independent interests.

You may find that people offer you conflicting advice and opinions about your duties and the patient's condition. You should try to build up a network of people you trust, based on your professional support team who know the patient's case in detail. Further support can be gained from joining an organization such as the Chest, Heart and Stroke Association

105

(CHSA): among their other activities, they support a national network of local clubs where carers and stroke victims can meet to share their experiences and enjoy socializing together. If there is no local group at a convenient distance from you, you could ask your therapist to put you in touch with other carers and patients, so that you can form your own support group, even on a very informal basis.

When you look after someone who is even only partly disabled, there is always a risk that you become so engrossed in his problems and needs that you forget to look after yourself. This can exhaust you, both physically and emotionally, which undermines your efforts to help the patient, so that you are both likely to end up suffering more.

Any significant stroke or head injury which happens to a person within a marriage, friendship or family situation alters your possible future plans as well as your day-to-day life. While the patient is suffering the frustrations and discomforts of being ill, you are likely to be worried about the long-term prospects of his recovery, how long it might take, or indeed whether he will recover at all. You may find it difficult and depressing to envisage the future with this uncertainty, especially if you have, for example, made plans for your mutual life right up to retirement stage. Shorter-term planning is inevitably affected. A young couple may have to shelve plans to have a baby, at least for the moment. You may have worries about whether the patient can return to work, or how you can plan future holidays for yourself or the family.

On a day-to-day level, you may find yourself with responsibilities you did not have previously, such as organizing the household accounts and paying the bills. Perhaps the patient always made the key decisions in the home, or you may have taken those decisions together, whereas you might now find yourself having to make the decisions for the patient, yourself and other members of the family. If you are looking after ageing relatives, or if you have young children, looking after an adult disabled dependant as well can add a heavy burden to an already crowded day. If the family finances have been badly affected by the patient's stroke, you may have to go to work as well as making provision for caring for the patient. If he was the sole breadwinner, you may have to go out to work for the first time.

You must not underestimate how much practical, physical and emotional strain this situation creates for you. You may have time to prepare for it while the patient is in hospital, but the reality is still likely to hit you hard when he comes home. If you can, you should try to work out in advance what the patient needs for his practical comfort; how you are going to arrange his living quarters and his access to the bathroom and toilet; and how he is going to occupy his time. At the same time, you should try to think ahead about your financial situation. You must take every opportunity to discuss the practical problems with your doctor and the social workers, occupational therapists and physiotherapists, to take advantage of their experience of dealing with similar situations, and to let them know if there are any particular difficulties you think you might be facing.

Emotional aspects may be harder to cope with, as they are harder to share. If you were close to the patient before his stroke, and were used to showing him affection by touching and kissing him, and if you still feel the same warmth for him despite his illness, you can help his morale greatly by continuing to behave as before, even if he seems not to respond. If you had a sexual relationship before, there is no reason not to continue, if the patient shows interest. The sensation of the genital organs is normally unaffected by a stroke, for instance, and having intercourse is not dangerous for the patient's blood pressure. You can talk to specially trained counsellors about any sexual problems: SPOD (Sexual Problems of the Disabled) is an organization offering advice on the emotional and physical aspects of resuming (or starting) a close relationship with a physically handicapped person.

However, if you feel repulsed by the physical changes caused by the patient's illness, you should still try to behave gently and affectionately towards him. If you feel you cannot do this, or if your relationship before the stroke or head injury was hostile anyway, you should discuss this problem with the doctor before undertaking the responsibility of looking after the patient. If you feel you have to make decisions such as leaving the patient or getting a divorce, you should discuss the prospects within the whole family as well so that communally you can come to the best solution for all concerned. You may find it helpful to contact RELATE, an organization of trained marriage guidance counsellors with a special interest in the problems of the disabled. They have many local branches, so you can check in your local telephone directory whether there is one near you.

The patient's attitude to you and other people around him can change dramatically because of his stroke or head injury. He may suffer a severe personality change from which he might not recover. His perceptual difficulties may make it impossible for him to recognize you and his immediate family or your relationship with him. In some cases the patient recovers from this state, and relates to his family as before. In other cases he remains cut off, although he may then recover well enough physically and mentally to start a new life, perhaps even setting up home with someone else and taking on a new job.

If the patient has changed a lot in his attitudes, you should bide your time at first, if you can, in case he does recover to become as before. Head-injured patients, especially, can be aggressive in the first stages of their recovery. They may also show inappropriate behaviour, which should be treated by a behaviour modification programme worked out by the therapist and the psychologist. The carer is vital for re-inforcing the programme: when the patient behaves correctly, he is rewarded with praise, whereas his bad behaviour is 'punished' by being ignored. The carer has to refuse to respond to shouting or aggressiveness or any other kind of unacceptable behaviour, to prevent it from becoming a source of attention for the patient. The carer has to issue the command 'No!' if the patient behaves badly. If this fails, the carer should leave the room, or take the patient into another room where he will be alone for a time.

Emotional lability, in which the patient responds with exaggerated emotions, for instance bursting into tears without any real reason, is often a problem for stroke and head-injured patients. An even more embarrassing version of this is reversed emotional lability, in which the patient responds to a situation with the opposite emotion from normal. For instance, he might burst out laughing on being told of a tragedy, or cry at joyful news. This is usually not because of any lack of understanding of what has been said, but simply because he has lost the normal control of his emotions. The problem usually gets better gradually, but the patient may be left with a residual tendency to respond oddly in certain situations. This usually lasts longest in patients with speech problems. It can sometimes be difficult to determine whether the patient is ill-tempered and perhaps foul-mouthed towards you because of the immediate effects of his illness and the frustration he feels, especially if he cannot speak normally, or whether it is part of a personality change which is going to last indefinitely. Some patients with severe behaviour problems, especially as the result of head injury, may have to be admitted to special treatment units for behaviour modification therapy. If the situation lasts for a long time with no sign of improvement, you should discuss the future very carefully with the doctor or hospital specialist, rather than trying to cope in a hopeless situation which cannot resolve itself.

Even if you are coping well enough overall, you may sometimes be provoked into anger against the patient, either because of his behaviour, or because of your mutual frustration at the situation his illness has created. You may even feel like hitting him. If you reach this stage, you will probably feel guilty about it, which adds to your own discomfort. What you should recognize is that it is a warning sign that you have been doing too much, and that you need to get away from the patient, at least for short periods in the day, if not for some days or weeks. The patient may be too dependent on you and too demanding. He may use a type of emotional blackmail against you and other people close to him, by constantly demanding attention but refusing to allow other people to perform necessary chores for him, on the grounds that 'you do it better'. Rather like a spoilt child, he can force you into feeling that his survival depends on your constant presence and care.

You should try to look at the situation objectively and philosophically, and, if you can, keep a sense of humour. In fact, it is better for both of you if the patient is looked after by several people rather than yourself alone, even if you are not at work and could be with him all day every day. The social services may be able to provide help to reduce your burden. Although the patient may feel more comfortable with you because of your familiarity, you can delegate everyday tasks such as taking the patient to the toilet, or helping him to eat, provided that you make sure the helpers understand how to treat the patient gently, and how to help him position himself correctly in order to control his spasticity. You can teach other members of your family how to take care of the patient in this basic way, or professional 'babysitters' who can come in to spend a few hours with the patient so that you can get away. If they learn how to handle the patient with the same care that you have learned from the physiotherapists, occupational therapists and nurses, the patient will be perfectly safe. If necessary, you can ask the professionals to teach your helpers, to be absolutely sure they learn how to handle the patient accurately.

You need to pace yourself, so that you do not get carried away by the never-ending tasks that could fill your day with frenetic activity. It is all too easy to sacrifice every waking moment to the duties of running the house and looking after the physical needs of the patient and other members of the family. Even then, you might still finish each day feeling guilty about the many chores which inevitably remain undone. In order to maintain a proper balance in your life, you must be prepared to allocate some time to yourself each day. If you cannot organize people to come into your home to look after the patient, he may be able to attend a local Day Centre run by the Local Authority. In your free time, you might go to the hairdresser or beautician regularly, work out in a gymnasium, do a sport, go swimming, go out to films, concerts, shows or restaurants, visit friends, take up a new hobby, take evening classes, or join a social club. If you feel specially stressed, you could go to relaxation classes, or ask your doctor to arrange counselling for you. You might prefer simply to sit alone in a separate room and listen to music or read a book. Time spent on yourself in this way will also benefit the patient: if you keep yourself physically fit and mentally alert, you will be better able to offer him worthwhile emotional support, and you will find your situation less draining.

A longer holiday period away from each other is also valuable if you are looking after the patient full-time. You may be able to arrange *respite care* in a recognized rehabilitation unit, where the patient will receive rehabilitation treatment as well as being looked after. Treatment may also be available in a Young Chronic Sick Unit or, for the over-65s, in a Geriatric Unit in a hospital. Otherwise, the patient might spend some time in a private nursing home, possibly paid for by the State. Usually the patient is taken into one of these units for a specified period such as a fortnight, but the time allocated might be indefinite in an emergency, for instance if the carer is ill. The patient is admitted to one of these units in order to allow the carer the freedom to go away on holiday, as it is well recognized that carers need a proper break at intervals, so you should not feel guilty about taking advantage of the opportunity.

Your reward, as carer, is knowing that you have done your best to make the patient comfortable and happy, and to help him through the recovery process from his illness, however long it takes. You should always remember that you can only look after the patient successfully if you also look after yourself.

Checklist for the carer

- Always remember that controlling the patient's spasticity is a 24-hour-a-day job, and you have to help the patient to achieve this.
- Learn the correct methods of handling and positioning the patient to help him control his spasticity.
- Do not let the patient smoke, if possible.
- Check that he takes any medicines prescribed for him correctly. Get the repeat prescriptions in time so that he is never left without.
- Make sure the patient has a good diet.
- Make sure he drinks enough fluids, but not too much tea or coffee.
- Learn the easiest and most efficient ways of handling the patient, so that you can help him move about without hurting yourself or wasting energy.
- Let the patient act for himself when he can, provided

that he performs the movements correctly and without increasing his spasticity.

- Be patient if he moves or speaks slowly: give him time and encourage him to express himself.
- Never ask or expect the patient to perform actions that his physiotherapist considers are too hard for him.
- Encourage the patient to do the types of activities recommended for him, and try to prevent him from sitting idly, or gazing at the television.
- Stimulate him to activity, but don't push him too hard.
- Don't undermine the patient's confidence by accusing him of not trying when he cannot fulfil a task.
- Try to avoid shouting at him or upsetting him emotionally.
- Set aside time to sit with the patient to relax and talk.
- Encourage him to socialize with family and friends.
- Let him rest if he becomes tired or frustrated.
- Let him get used to being looked after by other people, but make sure they understand how he should sit and move.
- Once he is safe, let him spend some time alone.
- Take him out of the house as soon as possible, and encourage him to go out alone when he is safe to do so.
- Spare yourself: allow yourself some time away from the patient each day, if possible, and organize longer breaks for holidays at intervals.
- Use the expertise and facilities of your local authorities and voluntary services for practical help, advice and social activities.
- Think positively, and encourage the patient to be optimistic.
- Encourage the patient to go back to work, at least part-time, if this is possible.
- If you experience difficulties with any aspect of the patient's care, ask the relevant specialist from your rehabilitation team what you should do.

7
Physiotherapy Treatment

Physiotherapy treatment is vital for the patient's progress and physical recovery. Skilled treatment for the hemiplegic patient is very specialized, and there is no viable substitute for it. Everyone involved in caring for the patient has to learn some of the techniques of handling and positioning him, in order to provide continuity. However, these elements of care should not be confused with the treatment methods themselves, and there are clear delineations between the various professional practitioners. While good co-operation from the nursing and medical practitioners speeds up the rehabilitation process, only the chartered or fully qualified physiotherapist with specialist training in the treatment of hemiplegic patients is equipped to provide a total programme of rehabilitation, based on an individual assessment of the patient's limitations and potential. Although the ultimate goal of rehabilitation is for the patient to be able to walk and function independently, not all patients can be expected to recover fully. However, virtually all patients can benefit from rehabilitation and learn to do at least a little for themselves, which alleviates some of the burden on the carer. There is no time limit on the patient's capacity for physical recovery, although an experienced physiotherapist usually knows within the first few weeks of starting treatment how quick or slow a hemiplegic patient's physical recovery is likely to be. Many patients go on improving their physical abilities for years after their stroke or head injury, if they continue to have skilled rehabilitation guidance.

The primary aim of modern physiotherapy treatment is to re-educate normal movement. In order to do this, the physiotherapist has to understand what normal movement is. The principle underlying this treatment method is the certainty that the central nervous system is capable of recovering function despite being damaged: any lesion in the brain, such as a blood clot, only interferes with one part of the brain, while other parts of the brain, plus the spinal cord, are left undamaged. The capacity of the central nervous system to recover function is technically called *neuroplasticity*. However, recovery does not usually happen by itself. The brain needs information which provides the experience of controlled movements, in order to respond with the ability to produce the same movement control. The information required is proprioceptive: it has to provide a kind of internal sensation or perception in order to activate the correct response. The physiotherapist has to analyse what kind of proprioceptive information the patient needs in order to relearn how to move normally, and this is different for every patient. Then she has to work out how to deliver this information to the patient in the most effective way. This is how the physiotherapist directs the recovery of the central nervous system.

The patient's affected side should work again with proper co-ordination within the whole body system. A brain lesion or injury usually causes some measure of spasticity, which is an interference factor preventing normal movement. The central nervous system adapts towards the spasticity, allowing it to dominate all the patient's movements, if it is not carefully controlled. The patient may try to use his 'good' side to compensate for the affected side of his body which he cannot move at will. But this overworks the undamaged parts, resulting in increased spasticity. Spasticity can also cause pain anywhere in the hemiplegic side: the pain may occur when associated reactions happen, for instance when the patient is asleep, or when he is moving without proper control. The physiotherapist has to counteract the effect of spasticity and its concomitant associated reactions through skilful handling, controlling and positioning of the patient's body parts. By creating favourable situations and environments in this way, the physiotherapist makes it possible for the patient to move actively and specifically without effort. When the patient's spasticity is controlled, he will no longer experience any pain.

This kind of treatment is always dynamic, never passive, and the patient is totally actively involved in it. If you watch the treatment sessions, you may sometimes think that the patient is not taking any active role in initiating movements, whereas the physiotherapist seems to be doing the movements for him. This is a technique designed to teach the patient how to follow a movement, adapt to a change of posture and cope with different situations without producing spasticity through making too much effort. He is in fact participating by following the physiotherapist's instructions and relaxing into the required movements. He has to be able to reduce the tension (technically *tonus*) in his muscles before he can make controlled movements. The background to active movement is the patient's control of his posture, and his ability to balance upright against the effect of gravity. Once he has this control, he can progress to making *selective movements*. These are more complex isolated actions performed by only one part of the body, such as bending a knee, bringing one hand to the mouth, or using the fingers individually as in pointing, or picking up objects.

The physiotherapist's role

The physiotherapist is motivator and facilitator, inspiring and encouraging the patient to do what he can at every stage. Each stage involves goals for the patient: while they have to be progressive, they should always be attainable so that the patient remains well motivated, and avoids depression. The physiotherapist has to have enthusiasm for the task she and the patient are undertaking. Although she sets the goals for him to achieve, in fact success depends on the mutual effort of the physiotherapist and the patient. If the physiotherapist sets the correct goals, they will be achieved, but she has to recognize that each patient reacts differently to rehabilitation, depending on a variety of factors. Some patients begin to recover their ability to balance and to use their limbs fully within two to three weeks, whereas others may take months or years to reach their full potential, especially if they have perceptual problems and severe spasticity. The physiotherapist has to be encouraging at all times, but this stops short of praising the patient when he has not achieved a required movement. Appropriate feedback is vital in the patient's relearning process, so he receives praise only when it is deserved: if he fails in any way, the physiotherapist remains encouraging and positive about it, but shows him how and why he went wrong, or she may simply leave that task for the moment and return to it later, when the patient can concentrate and get it right.

One important goal for the patient is walking, but he has to be ready before he tries. If he cannot balance and control his movements, it is no use for him to try to practise 'walking' with the help of therapists or nurses. It would amount to no more than the patient being dragged around with maximum support, using his unaffected side to try to keep up, and holding on to his helpers for dear life. He would inevitably be frightened by the experience, because he would know that he cannot yet expect to walk safely. As a learning experience, early walking without movement control does not contribute any kind of useful information to the patient's brain, so it is not a relevant exercise for the patient to build his movement progression on. This is why the patient is no longer given a tripod or quadrupod and taught to walk by using his unaffected side and leaning heavily on his support. This 'compensation' method of walking may seem to get the patient on his feet more quickly than the modern method, but it leaves him overusing his unaffected side, therefore he is constantly increasing and fighting against his spasticity. This is not only likely to be painful for him, but it undermines his stability, so that he can only walk slowly, with constant concentration, and he is much more likely to fall over if he has to change direction or if he is distracted.

Planning the treatment programme

The sequence of modern physiotherapy treatment normally follows a pattern: the patient has to recover his ability to balance first and foremost; then he has to recover his ability to transfer his weight from side to side; standing balance is the next stage, accompanied by the ability to sit down from standing up, and to stand up from sitting; selective movements using the affected arm and leg come next; then he learns to make steps, followed by walking; function in the upper limb (arm) and controlling it in order to make selective movements against gravity happens at a late stage; the final rehabilitation task is to regain functional, detailed movements in the affected hand and foot. This sequence is not a rigid stereotyped order. Many of the different parts of the rehabilitation programme are done in parallel, both within single treatment sessions and in the overall programme. The rehabilitation programme is planned around each of these aspects in relation to the patient's specific needs.

In order to set out an appropriate treatment plan, the physiotherapist has to understand normal movement, and how brain damage interferes with it. She has to know how to deliver appropriate information to the patient, to overcome the neurological deficit which is the result of the brain damage, and to help him react in the way she wishes by producing carefully controlled movements. Through her handling techniques she has to be able to control and inhibit the abnormal tonus or tension in the patient's affected muscles. There are certain areas of the body which can initiate movement patterns, if they are held and moved in certain ways, taking into account the effect of gravity on them. These are called *key points of control*. The main key points are the patient's head, shoulder girdle, spine and pelvis. By handling the key points with different speeds and rhythms, the physiotherapist can change the patient's body reactions, especially in relation to automatic spastic responses. Therefore, she often guides the patient by placing her hand on his chest, or both hands behind his shoulders or on his hip bones below his waist. The physiotherapist must be able to assess the patient's needs, both overall and from session to session, in order to define an effective rehabilitation programme and to set him realistic goals. It is also important that the physiotherapist should explain each part of the rehabilitation process to you the carer, teach you how you can help, and guide both you and the patient through each stage (and any setbacks).

What if treatment does not seem to be working?

If you feel the patient is making no progress at all, you should ask the physiotherapist if this is so, and why. In the normal way, there should be some change for the better in the patient's condition, so if weeks pass and the patient seems static, you need to know why. The physiotherapist may be able to point out changes which you have not noticed, but which show the patient has progressed adequately. Otherwise, there may be good reasons why he has not advanced, perhaps because he has been ill or over-tired. However, if it seems that the physiotherapist is not treating the patient effectively, you should ask whether, perhaps, he might be assessed and treated by a more senior physiotherapist, if he is attending a hospital department. If none is available, it may be possible to arrange for a specialist physiotherapist to visit the hospital department to see the patient and suggest appropriate treatment lines to the physiotherapist there. Otherwise, the patient might be transferred to a specialist Stroke Unit or have a private consultation with a specialist physiotherapist. If you can afford private treatment, or you have medical insurance cover to pay for it, you may prefer to take on a full treatment programme with the specialist physiotherapist. Otherwise, your hospital physiotherapist may be willing to see the specialist with you, for guidance which she can then put into practice herself. If the patient has been seeing a physiotherapist privately, it still may be necessary to involve a second, specialist physiotherapist, if the patient stops progressing.

If you do change practitioners, it is vital for good communication to be maintained between the physiotherapists involved, and with the patient's family doctor. The patient may not like the idea of changing, having got used to a particular physiotherapist, but if the change is made sensitively, the benefit of seeing a specialist will soon be evident, and he will adjust to the new situation.

Organizing the treatment sessions

When a specialist physiotherapist organizes a treatment session, every movement done by both patient and therapist has a purpose. Out-patient treatment may be done in a hospital, clinic, private practice or at the patient's home. In every case the physiotherapist tries to make sure the environment is right for the patient. The room has to be warm. Many patients find it difficult to concentrate in a noisy room, and are easily distracted, so the physiotherapist tries to reduce unnecessary noise. If the treatment sessions take place in a large gymnasium, for instance, the physiotherapist will screen off a section of the space for greater privacy, and so that the patient is not distracted by seeing what is going on around him. The session will be timed not to coincide with noisy exercise classes to music. If the sessions are done in the home, family or friends will be asked to be reasonably quiet, and not to turn the radio or television up, or have noisy conversations.

The physiotherapist needs at least one plinth (treatment couch), which, at about 40 inches (about 1 metre), is wider than a manipulation couch, which is usually about 24 inches (60 cm) wide. In many specialist centres two plinths may be available in the treatment room for treating a single patient. The treatment plinths are usually electrically operated, so that the physiotherapist can adjust the height easily while still supporting the patient, when necessary. For home treatments, the physiotherapist may carry a folding board to place over the patient's bed for a firm surface. Portable treatment couches are usually too narrow and lightweight for treating a hemiplegic patient. When the patient is having long-term treatment at home, it is often worthwhile for him to invest in his own treatment plinth, if he can afford it, and if there is space for it. The physiotherapist usually has several pillows available to support the patient, plus a wedge cushion, which is a foam support measuring about 2 feet (60 cm) long, $2\frac{1}{2}$ feet (76 cm) wide, 6 inches (15 cm) deep at the top, tapering down lengthwise to form the wedge shape. There may also be gymnastic balls of various sizes: these are like beach balls, but are made of extra strong plastic.

The physiotherapist may need the help of a second therapist, especially for the head-injured patient or the patient who has had a severe stroke. In the home she may ask the carer to perform the tasks of the assistant therapist. The patient with perceptual problems may be treated by the physiotherapist and the occupational therapist simultaneously, to help his overall awareness. The patient is expected to be suitably dressed for treatment: men usually wear comfortable, loose-fitting shorts, with adequate underpants underneath, while females wear shorts plus a camisole top, or a sleeveless vest with a comfortable brassière underneath it. Patients are usually barefoot, unless there is some special reason why they need shoes. A thin exercise mat is usually used for treatments where the foot touches the floor, to provide a secure and cushioned surface. The mat prevents the hemiplegic foot from being over-stimulated by contact with a cold floor.

Treatment techniques

Every patient is treated according to his specific needs, and every physiotherapist treats her patients individually, so there is enormous variation in the ways different physiotherapists treat different patients. You will not necessarily see your physiotherapist doing exactly the treatment techniques described below: she may use some of these techniques plus others she has devised herself, or she may use a completely different method. It is important for you to understand what the physiotherapist does, so that you can follow any instructions the physiotherapist gives you for remedial work at home, and can appreciate the patient's progress. You should never be afraid to ask the physiotherapist to explain what she is doing. The treatment techniques we describe are not a treatment programme as such: they are examples of what you might see the patient doing, with explanations of what the physiotherapist is trying to achieve, and how the patient should respond.

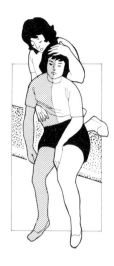

Balance practice: the physiotherapist moves the patient away from the upright position, and the patient returns to upright using the trunk and pelvis.

Treatments with the patient sitting

When the patient sits on the side of the plinth for treatment, the height of the plinth is selected according to the work to be done. If the patient has poor balance, he sits well supported on the plinth, with his feet flat on the floor. He may start sitting like this in preparation for moving into the supine lying position (on his back) or, more rarely, into the prone lying position on his stomach. Most of the work will concentrate on reducing his associated reactions, if these are strong and the patient's balance is poor. If he is to practise standing up, the plinth height may be raised, so that he is perched on the edge with his legs fairly straight: this reduces the support under his seat, but makes it easier for him to stand. The physiotherapist may sit or stand in front of the patient, or may kneel on the plinth behind him, according to the type of guidance she intends to give him.

With the patient fully supported, the physiotherapist may help him to do controlled movements with his pelvis: she places her hands on his hip bones, just below his waist and guides the pelvis in forward and backward movements. The patient may then progress to moving forwards and backwards using his seat muscles. This is part of learning to balance

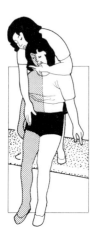

The patient is brought into the standing position, with the physiotherapist controlling the patient's head and pelvis.

successfully with the trunk well controlled, and without allowing associated reactions to distort the shoulder girdle or leg.

As a preparation for standing, the physiotherapist may place a large gymnastic ball on a table or second plinth in front of the patient. The patient places his arms on top of the ball, and is guided in a forward-backward rocking movement, using the ball as a kind of roller. This helps the patient to control his trunk movements symmetrically: he is guided into extending his trunk, stretching upwards, as he goes forwards, and then flexing (bending) the trunk as he comes backwards. These movements are similar to the normal rotations of the pelvis when you stand up, so the patient is practising them in order not to jerk upwards awkwardly or sideways as he stands, as this would inevitably knock him off balance.

With the plinth raised, and the patient sitting forwards on the side of it, he may practise similar controlled movements for the pelvis, or the physiotherapist might mobilize the patient's shoulder girdle to reduce any spasticity. The physiotherapist may also use this high sitting position to desensitize the patient's foot, especially if he has a strong positive supporting reaction (see p. 13). If the patient has a positive supporting reaction, the physiotherapist places his

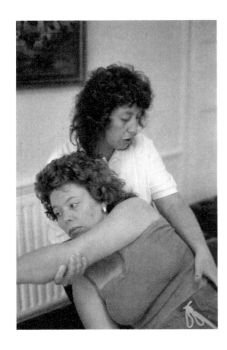

The physiotherapist controls the patient's pelvis during rotation movements to loosen the trunk and shoulder girdle.

foot carefully towards the floor, grading the pressure it receives in order to reduce the automatic reaction of pushing down as soon as it makes contact. In some patients there is a flexor reaction which makes the patient draw his foot away from the floor on contact. In this case, the physiotherapist gives the sole of the foot gently graded stretching as it is placed to the floor. When the patient can stand up success-fully, without incurring any associated reactions in the arm, trunk or leg, he may practise standing on the hemiplegic leg with the normal leg off the floor, resting on a stool. The physiotherapist controls the patient's balance reactions by maintaining control of the patient's hip and knee.

Advanced work for the hemiplegic arm may also be done with the patient sitting down. The physiotherapist usually starts by mobilizing the shoulder girdle, moving it passively in all directions, to make it perfectly pliable. She may also mobilize the hand, if it is tense and clenched. Then the patient's arms are placed on a table in front of him with the hands flat and fingers spread open. Holding the arms and

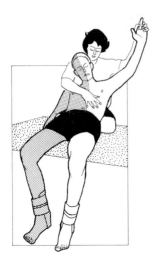

Guiding movement for the normal arm, to prevent the patient from over-using it. (The patient follows the movement, without pushing or pulling through his arm.)

hands still, the patient moves his seat sideways a little, then backwards and forwards, so that he is practising using his trunk without provoking any unwanted activity in his affected arm. The exercise is made harder by placing the arms wider apart on the table, and then by asking the patient to move the unaffected arm while keeping the hemiplegic hand still and relaxed in its position. The patient might roll a small ball slowly round the table with his normal arm, watching his hemiplegic arm in order to control any signs of unwanted reactions in it. In another movement pattern for arm and trunk control, the patient sits with his weight on his arms and moves his body, with the physiotherapist's guidance, so that his arms have to react to help his balance.

The later stages of arm control involve lifting the hemiplegic arm and controlling it in space while bending and straightening the elbow. These movements are done with both arms together at first, then alternately. When possible, the patient uses the hemiplegic hand to grasp objects or grip. This may be linked to functional activities, like lifting a cup to the mouth. At every stage, the physiotherapist checks that there is no spastic reaction arising from the movements being done: if necessary, she supports the shoulder girdle or elbow to help the desired movements to be made with full control.

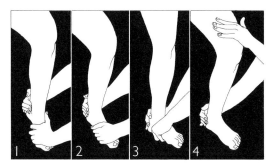

Desensitizing the positive supporting reaction; the physiotherapist concentrates on lengthening the sole of the foot and the Achilles tendon.

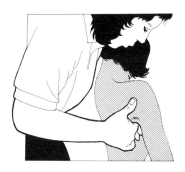

Mobilizing the shoulder girdle to release spasticity.

Treatments with the patient supine

One of the reasons for placing the patient lying on his back is to practise the movements needed for getting in and out of bed. He starts by sitting on the side of the plinth, and the physiotherapist may use mobilizing techniques to reduce any spasticity in the patient's trunk or arm. The patient then turns backwards and lifts the normal leg onto the plinth while the physiotherapist guides the hemiplegic leg as it too is lifted up. If the patient's spasticity increases as he goes through this sequence, the task is too difficult. He can only be

125

placed in the lying position for effective treatment purposes when he can balance well enough to be taken through this

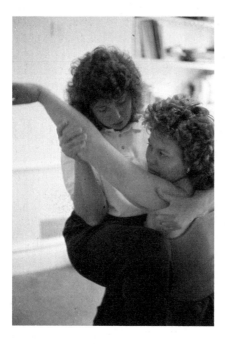

Mobilizing the hemiplegic shoulder and arm.

pattern of movements without increasing his spasticity.

When the patient lies on his back on the plinth, his head, shoulders and trunk are supported on a wedge cushion. If he were to lie flat, associated reactions might be stimulated by the pressure of the couch against the back of his head and upper back. He might also press back against the plinth when he tried to move his seat or legs. The wedge cushion has the further advantage of allowing the patient to see his legs without effort. If the physiotherapist wants to support the head and shoulder girdle even more, as a further barrier against spastic reactions, she may also place pillows under the hemiplegic side.

Once lying down, the patient may practise the movements needed to move into lying on his side and to get up out of bed: for these, he needs to be able to move his shoulder girdle, trunk and pelvis in isolation from each other. He may practise selective pelvic movements, in which he isolates the actions of tilting the pelvis backwards, forwards and sideways. He may practise lifting the pelvis in order to turn sideways, which is an essential pattern for turning over in bed. To help the patient gain control of his leg movements, the physiotherapist places the hemiplegic leg in certain positions, and asks the patient to maintain the position, checking

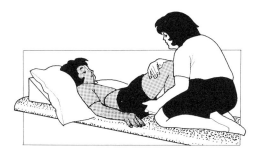

Selective, graded activity for the pelvis: the physiotherapist helps the patient to tilt the pelvis, while the patient follows the movements.

that he can do so without an increase in spasticity. He might practise controlled movements involving bending his knee, or bending and straightening his arm. More complicated patterns for the arm involve holding it straight and turned outwards at certain angles, where the physiotherapist has placed the arm, and then learning to move the arm between two positions.

The advantage of supine lying is that it allows the patient to work more easily, because the effect of gravity is reduced, and the patient feels safe because he is fully supported, so he can concentrate on perfect control of the selective movements in his limbs: this is an important stage in the preparation towards making steps, and ultimately to walking.

Treatments with the patient standing

The patient's first experiences of standing up, in the early stages after his stroke or head injury, aim to help his body regain the tonus needed to hold itself up against gravity (pp. 9, 115). In the following stages, treatment in standing concentrates on restoring his proper balance mechanisms, so that he can make better quality selective movements using his trunk, leg and arm.

The patient may have his arms and upper body supported on the treatment plinth as he stands facing it, while the physiotherapist sits on a second plinth behind him. The patient's plinth is high enough to support his arms comfortably at an angle of 90° to his body, while the second plinth is lower, so that the physiotherapist's feet are level with the patient's ankles, and her knees are roughly at the same height as his. The patient's arms are straight, and spread slightly apart. The physiotherapist, without shoes, places her feet over the patient's ankles to stabilize his feet, while her knees hold the outer sides of his lower legs, and her chest supports his seat. From this position, the patient comes backwards towards the physiotherapist, without moving his feet or arms, while she controls the movement of his pelvis. He practises tilting his pelvis in the correct pattern as he moves forwards and backwards, and he straightens and relaxes his knees as instructed and guided. This is a pattern to prepare for the movement of sitting down and standing up.

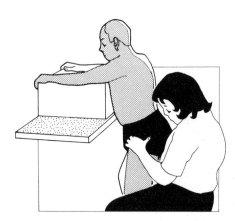

Working for control of the hemiplegic leg and the pelvis.

To help the patient transfer his weight from foot to foot, a side-to-side movement of the pelvis is performed, with the patient well stabilized by the plinth he is facing. When he has good balance standing up, the forward plinth may be lowered, and a gymnastic ball placed on it. The patient places both arms over the ball and rolls it forwards while extending

his seat backwards, and then selectively tilts his pelvis forwards and backwards, keeping his arms well in position over
the gymnastic ball. As the patient stands up, he practises
bringing the ball back towards him by bending his elbows
with good control.

For greater support, the plinth in front of the patient may
be lowered so that he can bend over it and rest his torso on
it, with his head turned to his normal side, and his arms
relaxed by his sides. The physiotherapist then guides the
patient in moving his hip, knee and foot selectively. This
position helps prevent the excessive trunk activity which
might happen when the patient is standing erect, and it helps
the patient to work from the very lowest part of the back, at
the pelvis.

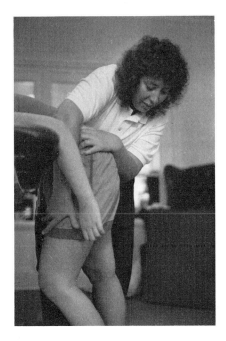

*Controlling the pelvis and
leg, with the patient's trunk
supported on the couch.*

Most of the work done with the patient standing up aims
to make his selective movements of better quality as preparation for making steps. Apart from isolating the movements
of pelvic tilting, knee bending and straightening, and foot
mobility, the patient is taught to transfer his weight onto one

leg, in order to be able to move the other leg away safely. The patient may stand on the hemiplegic leg, while the therapist moves his other foot into different positions, or asks him to move the foot. His first steps are taken by standing on the hemiplegic leg and moving the normal leg sideways. For this, the physiotherapist usually sits in front of the patient on a stool, in order to stabilize his pelvis and prevent him from folding in the middle. She helps the patient transfer his weight onto his hemiplegic leg, and then release his normal leg so that it can move freely sideways. Then the movement might be practised in the other direction, and the physiotherapist guides the hemiplegic hip and knee to move sideways with perfect control. The patient may then practise walking sideways in similar fashion round the plinth.

Once the physiotherapist is confident that the patient has gained full control of his hemiplegic leg while making sideways steps, she then guides him through a sequence of forward steps, starting with the normal leg, transferring the weight onto that leg to move the hemiplegic leg, and maintaining good control of the pelvis during the movement. Walking is taught through this detailed control of all the different aspects involved in making single steps. The physiotherapist provides careful feedback, helping the patient to learn how much to lift each leg, where to place the leg and the foot, and when to make each movement. If possible, the patient learns to walk without any support at all: if he learns to lean on a stick, tripod or quadrupod, his body balance is likely to become totally distorted, and he cannot learn the necessary body control to walk safely. However, if the patient has learned to make steps safely, but still tends to overuse his normal side, the physiotherapist may supply him with a high stick to help him to balance better. The stick is measured to the patient's normal hand held with the elbow bent to 90°. This is totally different to the measurement for a walking stick to help an injured hip or ankle, and on no account should the stick be shortened. The patient uses the high stick purely to help his balance, not to lean on. He may be taught to hold it with the crook of the handle turned away from him, and his thumb over the top of the handle, so that he does not grip the stick too hard.

At a very advanced stage of rehabilitation the patient prac-

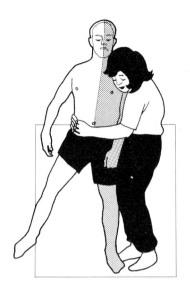

Balancing on the hemiplegic leg, practising weight transference.

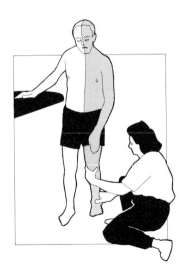

Working for selective movement in the knee, in preparation for walking.

tises controlling the hip swinging phase of walking, standing without support and maintaining his balance. He may also do complex movements for his arm, such as holding a long pole (like a broom handle) and moving it around and away from his body. The physiotherapist may hold the other end of the stick and direct the patient's movements, guiding the patient's arm and shoulder girdle so that they move in the correct sequence. With two long poles, the patient can practise synchronized arm movements. Another advanced pattern is for the physiotherapist to hold a cloth stretched between her hands: the patient holds the cloth in his hemiplegic hand and follows the movements as the physiotherapist takes the cloth in different directions, guiding the patient's arm around, forwards and backwards.

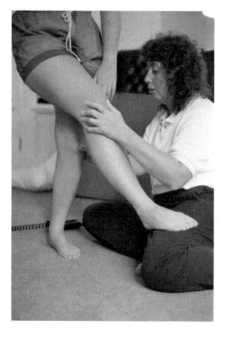

Advanced balance work, weight-bearing on the hemiplegic leg and moving the other across the body.

Treatments with the patient kneeling

When the patient has very good balance standing up, some movements may be practised kneeling down. These are usually related to functional activities. For instance, if the patient likes gardening, it is useful to be able to kneel to reach the ground, and he also has to be able to get up safely.

Kneeling down on a soft surface, the patient may practise trunk movements using the gymnastic ball to support his arms and shoulders, while the physiotherapist controls the balance of his pelvis. He can move forwards, rolling the ball forwards, and then come back almost to sit on his heels. When he has mastered this type of movement kneeling, more advanced work might involve sitting on his heels and then shifting his weight towards his hemiplegic side to practise controlling his arm and the side of his trunk while some of

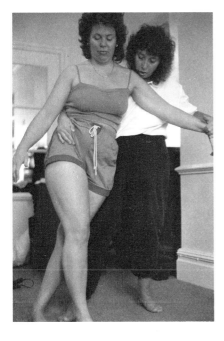

Making sideways steps, standing on the hemiplegic leg.

his bodyweight is transmitted from side to side.

Kneeling can also be used to help the patient get up from the floor; most patients are taught to do this once they can walk, in case they have a fall. If the patient can get into the kneeling position and then balance on one knee while bringing the other leg forward, so that he can lever himself onto a chair, he will feel confident that he can always get up, even if he is alone at home.

Treatments with the patient lying prone

Very few patients are treated in the prone lying position (on the stomach). The patient would have to have an almost normal trunk, without any associated reactions or increased spasticity as he was placed in the prone position on the plinth. He would be able to walk, and any work would be aiming to improve the quality of his walking, for instance if he had a slight limp. The prone position is not used for elderly patients or those with severe perceptual problems who might become severely disorientated, with increased flexor spasticity.

To get into position, the patient can start by sitting on the side of the plinth, going down gently to lie on his back, and then turning over. If he has had a very good recovery, he may get onto the plinth at a low height and kneel on all fours, and then be guided downwards to lie on his stomach. Lying prone, the patient's shoulder blade can be drawn well forward, so that he can practise selective movements with his arm, particularly turning (rotation) in different directions. He can also move his hip and knee into the extended position, with the physiotherapist carefully guiding his leg or controlling his foot. A very advanced movement is for the patient to lift the hemiplegic leg backwards and take it behind him, in order to roll over onto his back.

One of the practical tasks which may be taught to the patient in prone lying is how to get up from the floor. The patient may be placed on his stomach on the floor, and taught how to come up onto all fours, and then to kneel up, so that he can walk on his knees to a chair. Alternatively, the patient might be taught how to turn over onto his side and then onto his back, and shuffle towards the chair on his bottom.

'Homework'

The patient is not encouraged to practise walking at home until he can walk fairly normally, and without any increased spasticity in his arm. Walking without full control of the spasticity would only make it more difficult for the patient to gain that control in the longer term. On no account should the patient be allowed or encouraged to get himself around by dragging his foot and leaning on the furniture. Therefore, you will be asked to continue using the wheelchair to move the patient around until the physiotherapist is sure that he has reached the point where he can walk correctly and safely.

On the other hand, when the patient can stand up, he should use every opportunity to practise standing with proper balance. For instance, when he is wheeled to the toilet, he stands up in order to get into the wheelchair, and again to move onto the toilet, instead of being lifted or transferred. You have to make sure every time that the patient takes his weight as evenly as possible on both legs, with his trunk and arms in the right position. The physiotherapist may show you how to practise standing and balancing, with the patient supporting his arms at the correct height, perhaps on a chest of drawers. He may do the movements he has practised during physiotherapy sessions standing up, but supporting his whole trunk by leaning forwards over a cabinet or cupboard of suitable height. Once he has learned to take steps, he can practise these at home, perhaps using the kitchen fitted surfaces for support as he moves sideways in each direction. When he can make steps in the forward direction, you may be shown how he can use the lowest stair to practise stepping downwards while taking his weight through his hemiplegic leg and then through the normal leg. If he uses the banisters to do this, there should be rails on both sides of the stairs, to encourage symmetry of movement. If the patient's foot tends to twist as he stands on it, he may be given a special ankle support to help hold it comfortably in position.

As soon as the patient becomes familiar with the feelings he experiences during his physiotherapy treatment, he can practise pelvic movements at home, perhaps lying on the floor if he does not have his own plinth or a firm surface on his bed. He may use a gymnastics ball, resting on a table, to practise trunk movements, as he has done during his treatment sessions. You may also be shown how to guide his arm movements, if he has made a good enough recovery to practise these correctly.

'Homework' for the stroke or head-injured patient is not a question of 'doing exercises'. The aim is to reinforce the correct patterns of movement which the patient has experienced under the guidance of the physiotherapist. All the movements have to be done absolutely correctly, otherwise they make the patient's problems worse rather than better. The correct movements are an extension of the positioning which you have already been using to maintain the patient in the right body posture. The whole programme is a 24-hour-a-day rehabilitation concept, so it is vital that you understand what you and the patient should and should not be doing. If in doubt, ask your physiotherapist.

8
Case Studies

Dawn

Dawn was an attractive, lively girl who thoroughly enjoyed her work as a bank clerk, and whose social life centred on her favourite sports, hockey and tennis. One night, at the age of twenty-six, she was the victim of an appalling accident, when she was passenger in a sports car which ran out of control and somersaulted, landing upside down. The driver was killed instantly. Dawn's life was saved because two trained paramedics, travelling in the opposite direction in their private ambulance, noticed the sports car travelling at high speed, then realized it had crashed, and turned round to offer help at the scene. The paramedics resuscitated Dawn, who had stopped breathing, and they later received the Queen's Award for their prompt action. Dawn was taken immediately to the nearest hospital and put on a life-support machine in the Intensive Care Unit.

Dawn's parents learned of the accident some three hours later, went immediately to the hospital, and spent much of the rest of the night waiting for information. They were not encouraged to hope: it was likely that Dawn would die, but if she survived, the doctors could not be optimistic about her future condition. Dawn was in a deep coma, and was not responding to painful stimuli, although her pupils were not fixed. She had no obvious injuries apart from a broken shoulder blade. Initially, the doctors were not sure whether Dawn had suffered brain damage, so they arranged for Dawn to be transferred, still on the life-support machine, to a nearby hospital which could perform a CAT scan. Dawn's parents had to give their written permission for the transfer, which added to their anxieties about the situation.

The CAT scan apparently showed no damage to the brain, so it was something of a shock to the doctors as well as to Dawn's parents when she finally came round from the coma after about a week with a left hemiplegia. Her parents were told that Dawn had evidently suffered a stroke, and would probably recover to remain confined to a wheelchair. The better news was that her intelligence was unimpaired. Dawn's parents never understood at what stage Dawn had suffered the brain damage. They found this confusing, and, to a certain extent, it became a cause of resentment.

Dawn had little physiotherapy treatment while she was in hospital. Five months after the accident, her mother brought her to a specialist treatment centre in London. Her balance was very poor; she could not stand up on her own, because strong associated reactions would pull her left side over; her left Achilles tendon was extremely tight; her left shoulder was very painful; her arm was pulled into a bent position, with the hand tightly closed in a fist (flexor spasm); she could hardly sit up straight because of the severe spastic muscle pull on the left side of her body; her mother had to push Dawn everywhere in her wheelchair, and give her total nursing support.

Physiotherapy treatment was aimed at reducing Dawn's pain, lessening her spasticity, and trying to recover selective control of the movements in her left foot, ankle and knee. Dawn made good progress, and was soon able to stand up. Some eight months after the accident, she could balance. She was then able to walk with the help of a tall walking stick, and gradually improved to the stage of walking without a stick. This was a tremendous achievement, as she recovered little selective movement in her leg, and none in her left arm. Dawn spent fifteen months attending the centre. A physiotherapist from Dawn's area accompanied her to the centre on occasion to observe the specialist care she received. Dawn was then able to continue the same line of treatment with the physiotherapist locally.

During the long period of her recovery, Dawn understandably had bouts of severe depression, so at one stage she was referred to a clinical psychologist for counselling. The psychologist worked on the assumption that Dawn should prepare herself for a life of dependency on others, so he did not try to motivate her towards self-sufficiency. He referred Dawn to a neurosurgeon, who promised that he could operate to cure the spasticity which kept causing her muscles to tense up involuntarily. Dawn and her family were ecstatic. Fortunately, however, they knew enough about Dawn's condition to question the neurosurgeon closely when he described how Dawn would be fully conscious throughout the operation so that he could identify the damaged brain cells which were causing the spasticity, in order to destroy them. The surgeon was forced to admit that this operation would leave Dawn paralysed and wheelchair-bound for the rest of her life. The family was intensely upset, knowing that Dawn was potentially capable of physical independence, even though her spasticity made it so difficult for her to move normally. They all felt let down, and bitterly disappointed.

Most of Dawn's treatment was done privately, because she could not obtain adequate long-term treatment through the National Health Service. She had to make a claim against the insurers, because her friend had not had full cover for his sports car. The case dragged on, and the insurers made an offer of settlement. Dawn was advised that she might obtain more money if she went to court, but she felt that this would be too hard for her emotionally, even though she had no memory of the accident or indeed of the friend who had died. Therefore, three and a half years after the accident, Dawn accepted the amount offered, which was sufficient to pay back the £70,000 her father had spent on her treatment and a specially adapted car, and to provide her with an ongoing income to cover her living expenses.

The car was vital to Dawn's independence. It was adapted to be driven with one hand, and Dawn had to retake her driving test. It gave her the confidence to go out alone, even though walking was still difficult. Two years after the accident, Dawn was able to go shopping by car, walking such distances as were necessary. Another vital boost to Dawn's confidence and motivation was her introduction to the British 'Les Autres Sports', an organization which encouraged sports competitions for people with disabilities. Four years after her accident Dawn took up the javelin, shot and discus. Her only problem was her coach's lack of understanding of the problem of spasticity. Like many people, he believed controlling the spasticity was simply a matter of trying harder. He tried to persuade Dawn to 'take a run at her throws', despite her protestations that simply standing up and walking required constant mental effort on her part. She finally convinced him by trying to run into a throw, inevitably falling over and spraining her ankle. From then on he began to understand how difficult it is to control spastic muscles.

Five years after the accident, Dawn was making the best of her new life. She was training for the Paralympics. She was totally independent, being able to cook, wash, look after herself and her home, drive and walk where she needed to go, even though she could not use her left arm at all, and she had to work constantly to control the spasticity in the left side of her body. She decided not to go back to the bank, because they would have had to create a special job for her. She felt this would make her 'singled out', so she preferred to take on similar clerical work doing the accounts for her father's farming business. Her family remained totally supportive, and Dawn was beginning to enjoy a full social life again. Through her sport, she met her fiancé. They moved into a second floor flat, so Dawn now had to run her own home and travel to work each day. Away from the slightly protected environment of her parents' home, Dawn's return to independent life was complete.

Stanley

Stanley, an American writer resident in Britain for over twelve years, had a sudden stroke while out eating dinner with friends. He collapsed and became unconscious, so he was taken by ambulance to hospital, where he was admitted as an emergency. The doctors diagnosed that he had probably had a left-sided embolic stroke, and decided that he did not need surgery, so he was treated on the medical ward, where he remained for about seven months. He was forty years old.

It seemed likely that Stanley's stroke was connected with his lifestyle. He was very sociable, and enjoyed eating, drinking and smoking. He had often drunk to excess in alcoholic 'binges'. He had had a successful academic career at Cambridge University, where he had taken successive degrees leading up to his PhD. He had subsequently been very successful as a writer. At the time of his stroke, he had just finished a major biography, which had received critical acclaim, and he was researching for his next book.

The stroke had a devastating effect on Stanley's life. It had produced a massive oxygen lack in the left side of the brain, leaving Stanley with a right-sided hemiplegia, complete loss of speech and understanding of other people's words, and a total inability to read or write. His speech and comprehension problems made his initial rehabilitation treatment difficult. When he was discharged from the hospital, he continued to attend for rehabilitation treatment as an out-patient. However, his physiotherapist decided that he would progress better in a specialist unit, so he was transferred to the care of a specialist stroke treatment centre in London.

When he started attending the centre, he was still unable to speak, read or write, but his understanding of language was returning. He could understand commands if they were spoken directly and in short sentences. He could walk with the help of a nurse, but very slowly and with great difficulty, as his balance was extremely poor. Improving his balance was the priority for the first phase of his treatment, combined with establishing stability in his pelvis, re-educating selective movements in his leg, relieving his shoulder pain, and encouraging active movements in his right arm. He could not be left alone, as he was not safe. He needed help for all activities, such as getting in and out of bed or the bath. As he had lived alone before his stroke, he had to hire 24-hour nursing help, and a nurse accompanied him whenever he went out, which was initially only to attend for rehabilitation care.

Stanley also had to cope with epilepsy, a fairly common complication following a stroke. His fits, which happened mainly in the evening or at night, would leave him disorientated and make his balance poor again. His nursing care was gradually reduced as Stanley became more independent, but he continued to have a nurse in attendance overnight, when he was most likely to suffer the epileptic fits.

As Stanley continued to have problems travelling around, largely because of his speech difficulties, his family (in the United States) bought him a treatment plinth so that he could have physiotherapy care at home. They had control of all Stanley's finances, as he obviously could not manage them himself. For one year he had intensive treatment, with the physiotherapist and speech therapist attending his home three times a week. The physiotherapist showed all the nurses involved the handling methods for promoting Stanley's independent movement and for reducing the spasticity in his arm. Because of this continuity of care, Stanley learned to co-operate with all his carers, and his independence gradually increased. To help him communicate with people outside his own environment, a card system was devised by the physiotherapist, speech therapist and Stanley himself: a series of cards carried messages covering the various situations he would normally be in, with the explanation on the reverse side, 'My name is Stanley, and I am unable to communicate with you because I have had a stroke.'

About two years after his stroke, Stanley had achieved virtually full independence. With his inherent love of life, he started meeting people socially again, although he abstained from alcohol and cigarettes. His card message system gave him the freedom to go out alone and hail a taxi, showing the driver the appropriate card for the place he wanted to visit. He was even able to take his dog, his constant companion, to the local park in a panier on his three-wheeled cycle. His family gave him control of his own finances again, so that he had to resume making budgetary decisions in his everyday life, such as choosing between a meal at Claridges or a physiotherapy session.

Stanley's physical independence was achieved because he was young and motivated. He did not regain any ability to use his right arm, but he had minimal spasticity in it, and no pain. He managed to communicate to a certain extent through gestures and facial expressions, and he could put together short sentences. When his physical rehabilitation could be reduced to a maintenance level of about one session per fortnight, he started to attend the City University where the City Dysphasic Group organized special programmes in communication skills for adults who had suffered head injuries or strokes. He also had a computer at home with simple tailor-made programmes designed to help him find and match words.

The one single disappointment to Stanley during his recovery was his inability to read. He wanted to read books and the letters his many friends sent him. Some of this frustration was alleviated by listening: he used the Talking

Books service, through which tapes are delivered to and collected from the home, and his friends would talk to him at length on the telephone. When he wanted to make a phone call, he overcame the problem of looking up names and numbers by using a push-button telephone with a number memory.

Stanley had many friends, many long-standing, and some only recently met. Even after his stroke, he still had a charismatic presence, and people valued his company. He had a very strong character, and this helped him to live his life to the full, despite his disabilities. He died suddenly of another massive stroke three and a half years after his original illness. The crowd of mourners at his funeral bore witness to the affection and respect Stanley had earned through his life and work.

Rose

At the age of sixty-one, Rose had a massive cerebral haemorrhage. The illness was sudden: Rose had generally been very fit and healthy throughout her life, apart from a tendency to faint in warm, crowded rooms. Her husband Sid would recognize the warning signs when she turned pale and became anxious, and he would take her out of the room before she passed out.

Before her illness, Rose was a very sociable person, enjoying a full life with her husband Sid, who had retired two years previously. They lived in Central London. As a Jewish family, they lived a structured, close-knit life. Rose used to get up very early, at 5.30 a.m., in order to finish the household cleaning and ironing before her husband woke up. Before retirement, Rose and Sid had worked together very successfully in business, running hotels and gaming clubs. Rose was also a skilful card player, and for several years she was world champion at poker. She retired before her husband, but continued to run her household according to her strict routine, while enjoying more of her own social life. In the mornings, for instance, after finishing the household chores she might go shopping, and then have lunch with friends.

She and Sid also travelled a lot, and were generally very content with their lifestyle.

On the day she was taken ill, Rose had a severe headache, which became so bad that she called her doctor, who asked a neurologist to visit her immediately at home. The neurologist diagnosed a possible brain haemorrhage, and had Rose admitted to a specialist hospital in London. She was taken by car, and walked into the hospital. She was kept on bedrest, and an angiogram was taken which showed that there was blood seeping into the brain from aneurysms which Rose had in fact probably been born with, but which had not caused any problems previously. After a few days the surgeons opened her brain (craniotomy) from the right side, and clipped the aneurysms.

Rose's family was told that the operation was a matter of life-and-death, so they gave the surgeons permission, even though they were also warned that the operation could result in further bleeding and disability. Rose was not told this, for fear of destroying her morale. Unfortunately, during the operation, Rose did suffer further distress and bleeding into the brain, and was left with a very severe left hemiplegia. Afterwards, she felt very much let down by the family's decision, saying she would have preferred to die rather than live in such a disabled condition. Because she was physically worse after the operation than before it, Rose was convinced that the doctors had made a mistake, and for a long time she wanted to sue them.

After the operation, Rose remained in the hospital for four months. She was in a coma at first, and then she suffered complications because her blood pressure became unstable. She showed severe potential spasticity, so the physiotherapists took great care to prevent her from being twisted into deformity. She also developed thalamic pain syndrome, a special complication in stroke when the patient has suffered really severe brain trauma. The syndrome causes bizarre responses to any stimulus to the hemiplegic side, so Rose might feel very cold in very hot weather, for instance, or might perceive the lightest touch as extreme pain. She also suffered badly from perceptual problems, losing her normal awareness of her own body and of the people and objects around her. She was terrified that she might fall, and so used to fight off anyone who tried to move her, even when she was sitting down.

Rose was unable to do much when she was discharged from hospital after four months, but she assumed she would recover all of a sudden, because her illness had come on so suddenly. She was transferred from home to a private rehabilitation centre, but she was not happy there because she had little privacy, and her family could not travel to see her every day. She was expected to join in class work, but her pain and spasticity increased because of the physical efforts she was making, and because of her stress. After several months, Rose was still unable to do much for herself, and her physical condition was in fact worse. She was discharged from the rehabilitation centre, and returned to the original hospital for out-patient physiotherapy treatment.

The physiotherapists began the task of bringing Rose's spasticity under control, and, some fifteen months after the stroke, she was referred to a specialist stroke treatment centre not far from her home for intensive rehabilitation. She was still badly disabled, confined to a wheelchair, and unable to control her spasticity at all, even when she was sitting or lying down. Her left arm was locked to her side, because her shoulder was extremely painful. She would scream if anyone came near her left arm, and she cried at night, begging for painkillers. She was depressed and frustrated. Her family was understandably distressed at her problems, especially because they had been told that the situation would gradually get better, and in fact it had got progressively worse.

A hydrocortisone injection failed to relieve Rose's shoulder pain, but with physiotherapy treatment the pain gradually receded, and it was possible to lever the arm gently away from her side. Her trunk movements slowly became more controlled, so that Rose could begin to balance. She learned to stand up from sitting in a chair, and within two years she was able to walk short distances, even outside, with very little help. She was able to move safely from room to room in her house, and she could get up during the night to use her commode when necessary. She managed to cook again, and her depression eased as she achieved a measure of independence and joined in the family's social activities once more. Throughout her recovery, Rose's husband and children supported and encouraged her efforts.

Sadly, Rose suffered a major setback one day, when she had a *grand mal* epileptic fit. She had had a long treatment session, and then decided, possibly over-ambitiously, to visit her brother for tea, walking part of the way. She had the fit in the car on the way home, and she had to be taken to hospital for treatment. Following this, she retrogressed to the starting point of her rehabilitation, with severe spasticity in her arm and leg, and an obsessive fear of falling, even from her wheelchair. She had occasional epileptic fits after the first, and they so frightened Rose and her family that everyone became over-protective of her. Rose no longer wished to go out, nor could she tolerate being left on her own, so she became totally dependent on other people. She stopped trying to move herself voluntarily, and relied on nurses to move her arm and leg for her, so that their task was to ensure that she was always correctly positioned in relation to her spasticity, after they had performed the normal nursing duties of bathing her and helping her on and off the commode. When there was no nurse in attendance, for instance overnight, Sid would help Rose if she needed to move.

Rose's dependence led to a quick decline in her physical condition. She became increasingly deformed as the spasticity twisted her body uncontrolledly. Because she was not moving at all, she developed a weeping wound in her leg one day, and the circulation collapsed to the extent that she nearly had to have the leg amputated. A special foot-pump used twelve hours a day saved the situation, and Rose subsequently had to use the pump for at least an hour a day to prevent a recurrence of the problem. Most importantly, Rose had lost motivation to help herself and achieve progress, and no one around her could help restore it. She was constantly depressed. Physically, she was still capable of walking, but she would only walk with her physiotherapist, never with the nurses or her husband. Her life was restricted to sitting in a chair, with her telephone, television, books and refreshments close to her right hand. Her greatest frustration was being unable to run her family home, and she had lost confidence in her ability ever to do that again.

Her family remained supportive, despite the emotional load: they remained hopeful that Rose would one day regain the motivation to try to help herself, and therefore the people around her. They knew that physically Rose could do much more than she was willing to try, so they kept searching for the key that would restore her will to live without being, unnecessarily, a burden on others.

Guy

Aged sixteen, Guy was riding a borrowed motorbike when he fell off and hit his head. He was not wearing a crash helmet. He was knocked unconscious immediately, so an ambulance was called. His father was told about the accident, and he arrived at the scene quickly enough to accompany Guy to hospital in the ambulance. At the hospital Guy's reflexes were all right, and he did not seem to have any brain damage, so the doctors told his father that he just had concussion. They became worried later on when Guy's temperature went up dramatically, so he was transferred to a local major hospital. A brain scan showed extensive bleeding around the brain, and the specialists concluded that Guy had been suffering from internal bleeding since his accident on the previous day. He was treated as an emergency case, and given a tracheostomy. He was put on a ventilator under sedation, and was given drugs through a drip to take down the bleeding and swelling in his brain. Guy's parents asked if he would live, and were told that he would, but that the doctors would not know how much brain damage he might have suffered until he came out of the coma and regained consciousness. After several days on the intensive care unit, Guy, still unconscious, was transferred back to the original hospital closer to his home.

Two and a half weeks after the accident, he began to regain consciousness. When a nurse first saw him move around in his bed, she gave him a pencil and piece of paper: he wrote a note asking for his watch. He was taken off the ventilator, although he still had the tracheostomy and a catheter for his urine. He had a left hemiplegia, and was flaccid at first, although the flaccidity soon started changing to spasticity.

After a few weeks, he was transferred to a rehabilitation hospital, where he received physiotherapy treatment. Although his left arm showed no sign of recovery, he began to stand and make steps, and his speech improved day by day. After about eight weeks he was discharged home, although he was still confined to a wheelchair.

At this stage, Guy and his family felt abandoned by the medical profession. He was given no follow-up treatment to continue the progress he had made in the rehabilitation hospital. The neurosurgeon who had been in charge of Guy's case in the hospital would give them no help or advice, and neither did the doctors. The family spent over six months trying to find out where Guy could receive specialist treatment. The family doctor advised them to try a well-known rehabilitation unit, not realizing that it specialized in orthopaedic rather than neurological cases. The treatment he received there made him increasingly spastic. He joined in exercise classes to stretch and strengthen his muscles, and consequently became increasingly disabled. His left Achilles tendon became badly shortened, making it difficult for him to put his foot to the floor, and he had a strong positive supporting reaction in his foot. Therefore he walked very stiffly and awkwardly, swinging his leg out sideways in order to force it to go forwards. He also had epilepsy, suffering three or four major fits per year.

After a spell at the rehabilitation centre, Guy's parents realized it was a mistake, and tried to have him transferred to a specialist stroke rehabilitation centre in London, even though this was a long way from home. There was a long wait. He was finally accepted for treatment about eighteen months after his accident. Guy attended the specialist treatment centre at regular intervals, and he received treatment at home from a local physiotherapist who liaised with the specialists at the centre. When he started treatment, the positive supporting reaction in his foot was difficult to desensitize because he had learned to walk using the abnormal reaction when he was in the orthopaedic rehabilitation centre. His balance was still very poor. He could not use his arm at all, by himself, and his shoulder was very painful. He had very strong associated reactions in the arm whenever he moved at all.

In treatment, he was guided through intensive work for his shoulder girdle to release the spasticity. The physiotherapists also worked to relieve his shoulder pain and realign the joint. They helped him regain selective movements in his arm, and to control the grasp reflex in his hand. Concentrated work was done for Guy's pelvis and foot, to improve his standing balance. Then he worked on gaining better control of the movements in his left knee. Guy gradually improved, until he had minimal problems with spasticity in his arm, so that his arm no longer interfered with normal activities such as dressing. He still could not use the arm actively by himself, but it was no longer painful. About four years after his accident, Guy learned to stand on his hemiplegic leg without his toes flexing automatically, so that he could hold his balance while he lifted his other leg off the floor. His foot and leg movements improved immeasurably, and his walking gait became more normal as he learned to swing his leg in the right pattern.

Because of his accident, Guy missed the later stages of his school career. However, he took evening classes in some subjects, and started part-time work about three and a half years after the accident. He gradually took on full-time work in the same company, and gained three promotions within a year. By the age of twenty-one he had a managerial post in charge of fifteen people. Having been very active before the accident, Guy resumed sport as soon as he could. He learned to play golf one-handed, although he could also use a two-handed grip sometimes if he controlled the left hand carefully with the right. He played snooker one-handed, and swam. He could ride a tricycle without difficulty, and was aiming to progress to a bicycle with stabilizers. He could control his left arm on the handlebar when riding a push-bike, but he found he could not use an exercise bicycle because the effort involved automatically increased his spasticity beyond his control. Apart from work and sport, Guy also led a full social life.

In returning to a full and active life, Guy was helped very greatly by his family. Although his mother remained upset about the accident, and was naturally more protective of him, his father took the view that if Guy did not perceive himself as disabled, nobody else would, and this proved to be the case. Guy was always very close to his older sister, and after his accident she treated him consistently in the same way as she had before, which helped him to regain his normal social skills very quickly. Always an easy-going person, Guy had no difficulty in making friends in any situation. For his twenty-first birthday, five years after his accident, his parents threw a large party to celebrate his continuing enjoyment of life. His only regret was that he could not drive, because of his epilepsy. However, he took care to control it, monitoring his own drugs, and remained optimistic that this problem too would recede with time.

 ### *Esther*

At the age of thirty-four, Esther was twenty-nine weeks pregnant with her fifth child when she developed toxaemia associated with high blood pressure. She was admitted to hospital and the baby was induced because the doctors feared both Esther and the baby were in danger. Although weak, the baby was basically healthy, but she had to be kept in intensive care for the first few weeks. Esther was allowed home, although she had to return to the hospital every day to breast-feed the baby.

Both mother and baby appeared to be doing well, until, about six weeks after the birth, Esther suddenly felt ill. She was visiting her mother before going on to the hospital to feed the baby. Feeling that she could not move her left arm or leg, she sat down on the stairs. She remained conscious, but became increasingly disorientated, losing all awareness of where she was or what was happening to her. Her mother called Esther's husband over. He asked Esther to stand up, but she could not, so he and Esther's father carried her onto the settee where she could rest. The doctor came, and arranged for Esther to be re-admitted to the gynaecological ward of the hospital so that she could continue nursing the baby, if possible. The doctor did not tell the family that Esther had probably had a stroke, for fear of alarming them.

In hospital Esther had tests including a CAT scan and an angiogram, and the doctors concluded that Esther had suffered a stroke from a thrombus. They felt the probable cause was the long period of high blood pressure she had experienced before and after the birth of her child. Esther was treated with anti-coagulant drugs, and the doctors monitored her kidneys, which they feared might have been damaged as a complication of the toxaemia. The effects of Esther's stroke were not obvious at first, which made the doctors wonder if she had suffered a second stroke when they found later that she had a very severe left hemiplegia.

Esther spent seven weeks in hospital, with her baby, although she needed help to look after her. She had little memory of this period later on. She was discharged from hospital and went home, but was confined to a wheelchair, as she could not walk. She was unable to stand up, but could sit in a chair without losing her balance. To help her recovery, she was referred to a specialist rehabilitation centre for younger patients. She had intensive physiotherapy treatment every day on a one-to-one basis, and gradually recovered her balance, so that she could stand up and walk with some help. Her spasticity was severe, but her rehabilitation helped her to control it. She had no recovery in her arm at all. After two months Esther was allowed home for weekends, so she was able to join in her normal family life, particularly celebrating the Sabbath. The family were Orthodox Jews, so this was specially important for Esther. She was determined to get better, and after seven months she was discharged from in-patient treatment at the rehabilitation unit. She continued to attend the unit as an out-patient for more than six months, when the therapists felt they could not make any further progress.

The occupational therapist had asked Esther's husband to prepare a downstairs bathroom and toilet for Esther, as she thought she would never be able to go up and down stairs on her own. She also thought Esther would need a hoist to get in and out of the bath. Esther refused to think in these terms, and insisted that she would be able to manage in her home as it was. She was very determined, and very soon after her return home she was managing the stairs, and later she was able to use the bath without a hoist. As soon as she could, she resumed the normal pattern of her life, getting up at 7.30 a.m. to prepare breakfast for the older children and get them ready for school. Then she would dress the youngest child.

At first, she only worked on the household duties, especially the cooking. Once she had the confidence to walk outside, she would see the older children to the bus-stop and then perhaps go shopping or meet friends.

Esther's speech and understanding were not affected, but she was quite badly disabled. Two years after the stroke, Esther still had very severe associated reactions in her left arm, which interfered with her activities: the arm would always be in her way and never where it was needed. Her leg felt heavy and difficult to move. She could walk, but had to hold onto things for support. She was very afraid of taking weight through her left leg, and could only feel deep sensations on her left side, so that it was difficult for her to know where her arm and leg were in space. She also had severe perceptual problems and found it hard to recognize the different parts of her body or to know where objects were in relation to herself. Her left field of vision was impaired (technically *hemianopia*), so that she had to turn her head and use her right eye in order to see anything even slightly to the left of her. She sometimes felt depressed, and would ask her husband if he thought she would ever recover: he was always supportive. He had been told from the start that recovery would happen, but it might take some years, so he felt their hopes were realistic. Generally, Esther remained optimistic. She felt she could still continue to improve, so she decided to have further specialist physiotherapy treatment privately, under her medical insurance scheme.

The treatment concentrated on reducing Esther's spasticity in her left side, and training her not to over-use her right side. She did a lot of work in sitting at first, gaining the feeling of balancing onto her left side, and she was taught how to move her spine more normally. As she was already walking, she did more work in standing than she otherwise would have, to promote the feeling of taking weight through her left leg while keeping her spasticity under control. As she progressed, she began to learn how to correct her balance when she was displaced by the physiotherapist, so that her confidence in her balance on her left leg was increased. She had regular treatment sessions for the next two years, and was still making progress. Her left arm was now under control, staying loosely by her side as she used the other arm and moved around. She was even beginning to gain some active movement in it during the treatment sessions. Her beautician noticed when her left hand began to stay relaxed while she manicured Esther's fingernails. She could walk more normally, manage stairs and go out alone safely. She ran her house as previously, looking after the five children and her husband. She could go to the synagogue and to large shopping centres as before, without having to worry about coping with stairs or moving about in crowds.

Esther's biggest regret was the advice she received not to think of having any more children. The doctors were adamant that the risk of a further stroke was too great to justify another pregnancy. She felt her stroke was due to the fertility drugs she had taken before each pregnancy, rather than to the childbirth itself: for the fifth pregnancy she had received injections of the drugs for the first time. However, Esther always remained positive in her outlook: she wanted to walk normally, as before, and to be able to use her left hand. Above all, she wanted people not to think of her as disabled. Her family treated her as before, and she was prepared to continue working hard at her rehabilitation so that she could feel normal again, and be accepted by other people as such.

Miranda

When Miranda's car was involved in a head-on collision with a lorry in a narrow country lane, witnesses thought she was dead as she lay trapped in the wreck. She was twenty-three at the time, and was working for the same firm as her father, after finishing her Master's degree in History. She came from a happy, close-knit family. She had returned home to London after finishing her studies, and was just buying her first flat. She was a lively girl, with a full social life and many friends.

Miranda's life was probably saved by a young man who thought he saw her move, and so climbed into the car to clear her mouth of blood and do basic first-aid. Twenty minutes later a doctor arrived on the scene, part of a voluntary patrol of doctors who normally attended accidents on the nearby main motorway to London. Miranda was put on a drip, still trapped and unconscious. She was finally cut free after about an hour by the Fire Brigade and taken by ambulance to the nearest major hospital. She was put on a ventilator in intensive care, and her legs were put into traction, because she had broken both thigh bones.

Miranda's mother and father were informed as quickly as possible: her father was in the United States on business, and his company flew him back on Concorde so that he could accompany his wife to Miranda's bedside that evening. They found their daughter unconscious, her face badly cut, surrounded by the paraphernalia of intensive care. The hospital staff were kind and reassuring. Miranda's parents were allowed to stay in the hospital overnight, and the doctors and nurses took care of them at the same time as they were busy saving Miranda's life. The parents were given hope: Miranda would probably not die. But they were not led into false hopes: it was too early to tell how much she would recover, as the brain scan showed diffuse bleeding into the brain, denoting a very serious head injury.

After about ten days, the consultant neurologist gave Miranda's mother bad news, which she remembered as one of her worst moments. Miranda was so badly brain damaged that it was unlikely that she would ever make any significant recovery, so she was probably going to remain a 'vegetable', and would not be able to return to any kind of home life. However, the nursing staff were more positive, and they advised Miranda's mother to contact 'Headway', a self-help group founded by the parents of brain-damaged children in order to provide encouragement and practical advice to people in a similar position. Miranda's mother talked to them and read their literature, and was reassured by their descriptions and explanations of what was happening to Miranda. Not only did it help her to come to terms with the current situation, but it gave her hope that Miranda might recover, at least to some extent. She was supported in her optimism by her husband and their two younger daughters.

About two weeks after the accident, when Miranda's head injury was stabilized, the orthopaedic surgeon operated successfully to insert rods into Miranda's thigh bones, so that she could be moved safely. A week later she was transferred to a major London hospital close to home, where she could receive specialist treatment and rehabilitation. By this time she was developing very stiff joints through spastic pattern-ing, to the extent that her limbs were becoming severely distorted and fixed in *contractures*. A further brain scan showed that Miranda had swelling and pressure building up in her brain, so a shunt operation was performed to relieve it. Two days later Miranda received her first active physio-therapy treatment. Although she was still totally unre-sponsive, the physiotherapist sat her up on the edge of her bed. Miranda's mother started to keep a diary, to reassure herself on a day-to-day basis that Miranda was making pro-gress. At this stage Miranda was 'floppy' in her trunk and spastic in her limbs, so she had no control at all of her movements. She had a strong positive supporting reaction in her right foot, which made her foot jerk rigidly when it was touched, and she had a grasp reflex in her right hand, so that any contact made her clench it tightly. She was also unable to hold her head up, speak, open her mouth, or swallow, and she remained semi-comatose, as though she was asleep most of the time.

Her physiotherapist was optimistic, enthusiastic and ener-getic, which encouraged Miranda's mother. Miranda was put into the standing position on a tilt table, and she was placed in the sitting position with her head supported. The physiotherapy treatment was intensive: Miranda's arms, trunk and leg were all moved to reduce the spastic patterns and to stimulate normal responses, even though Miranda herself remained cut off from the world. The physiotherapist made Miranda a special plaster cast, called a *drop-out plaster* to encourage her arm to straighten without putting pressure on her elbow. Every day, the physiotherapist talked to Miranda and encouraged her, and showed her mother every tiny change she saw in Miranda's condition.

Nearly three months after her accident, Miranda was beginning to come out of the coma. She seemed to be aware of her surroundings and listening to what was said, even though she still seemed 'asleep'. She seemed to recognize her mother, and gradually learned to make gestures like waving goodbye when her mother left the ward. Careful desen-sitizing techniques for her mouth allowed her to open it. Her mother and the nurses gently tried to feed her each day until she could accept the food, and she gradually learned to chew and swallow. She was still incontinent, partly because she had had a painful pressure sore from a badly applied leg splint shortly after the accident. However, she gradually began to be able to sit and hold her head up, and she could just help to put her arm and head into clothes when she practised dressing. She could not speak, but learned to point to cards printed with 'Yes' and 'No' in response to questions. The hospital wanted her to have speech therapy, but could not provide it, so Miranda's parents paid for a private speech therapist to work with her. She began to nod and shake her head replying to questions. She learned to suck fluids through a straw, and to wipe her mouth gently with a tissue. Her mother was delighted when Miranda could open her mouth enough to let her mother brush her teeth.

Miranda's whole family gave her constant encouragement and support. They would often take her outside in her wheelchair, to give her a change from the hospital ward. She began to go home for one day a week, and the family invented new ways of making her aware. She began to recognize photographs, and to identify colours. She could even match colours to their names, and she started to use a word processor to write words in response to questions. She still could not speak, although she understood language and could use written words. She had a true *dysarthria*, or inability to produce sounds: her only sound was to cough, and her mother used to encourage her to make coughing noises so that she might activate her vocal cords.

Five months after the accident, Miranda was transferred to a specialist rehabilitation unit, as she no longer required full nursing care. She spent a year being treated there, going home at weekends. Her parents organized private physiotherapy sessions at home at the weekends, because they felt that the continuity was vital to maintain Miranda's progress. When Miranda was discharged from the rehabilitation unit, she went to stay in a sheltered residential unit for the weekdays, so that she could practise living as independently as possible, although help was available if needed. She continued to have specialist rehabilitation treatment three times a week, plus the private physiotherapy sessions at weekends. Miranda was issued with a standard wheelchair through the

National Health Service, but this was too basic for 'adventurous excursions', so her parents decided to buy a second, better wheelchair. They took advice from the Disabled Living Foundation Equipment Centre, and then had the chair specially made by an expert supplier. When at home, Miranda used one wheelchair upstairs and the other downstairs, so that her family did not have to keep carrying the chairs up and down.

Eighteen months after her accident Miranda was beginning to be able to speak relatively clearly. She was using a word processor to write letters and do a little work for her employers. She could also write by hand: fortunately she was left-handed, and her right hand was the worse affected by spasticity. She could dress and undress, stand up, move from her chair to her bed, and go to the toilet, provided there were adequate supporting rails. She could manage to walk down a long flight of stairs with the help of just one person. Her physiotherapists insisted that she should not use a walking aid such as a frame, although this might have given her more short-term independence of movement. If she learned to lean on a frame, she would undermine her control of her spasticity, and this would halt the continuing progress she was making in improving her balance. Her parents understood this and agreed, even though at this stage it meant more work for them when Miranda was at home. They encouraged Miranda to go out with her friends. She enjoyed going to restaurants and the theatre, and she also travelled abroad on short trips with her family.

Sometimes, Miranda would get depressed, remembering her life before her accident. However, she was also optimistic. She could not remember anything from six months before to about six months after the accident, but although her short-term memory was weak, it was improving all the time. She and her sister were each to buy a self-contained flat attached to their parents' home. She enjoyed choosing the furnishings and decorations for herself. She was looking forward to having her own place, and being able to cook and entertain again. Her optimism was justified by the fact that she was obviously improving physically all the time, even though progress was slow. Although Miranda's parents were understandably more protective of her following her accident, they were also determined to encourage her to live as full a life of her own as possible. They were grateful that they had enough money to cover necessary expenses to improve the quality of her life. They were also thankful that they followed the course of optimism recommended by the nurses and therapists who cared for Miranda.

Both Miranda's parents spent a lot of time with her, and were prepared to make sacrifices for her sake. Miranda's mother had been developing a new career for herself as her children had grown up, and she gave this up in order to look after Miranda. She was delighted that their combined efforts were producing the results they wanted, but she expressed her shock at some of the things she learned through the experience: 'I feel *strongly* that the stimulus of family and friends is vital – I have consciously used time with Miranda as learning time in all sorts of ways – forcing her memory to establish facts, making her make decisions, however small, watching physiotherapists closely so I could carry on their work when transferring Miranda, or helping her walk. Although I do understand that head-injured people can only learn at their own, probably very slow, pace, and that one mustn't confuse them with too many decisions, I feel that the input of therapy at her initial rehabilitation unit was totally inadequate. I think this was probably due to under-funding, and as it is one of the best units in the country it is a terrible indictment of how unimportant this area of medicine is held to be. When one sees the possible range of recovery/dependence it just seems desperately short-sighted not to push large resources into the first year of recovery at least, by which time a longer-term prognosis could probably be made. The State could only benefit in the long run. I really fear that if we had lived far from a major city Miranda would not be in any way as advanced, nor if we had been unable to afford extra specialized therapy by highly trained and committed therapists.'

Ike

Ike was a successful hairdresser in her late twenties, running a chain of hairdressing shops with her husband. She was six months pregnant when she had a stroke. She and her husband had been trying to have a baby for eight years, and she had taken fertility drugs during this period. Ike had suffered from very bad headaches throughout the pregnancy, but had not had high blood pressure. Three days before the stroke she felt slightly faint. The stroke happened suddenly, while she was dressing one morning. She collapsed unconscious on the floor, but came to quickly. She felt as though she was very drunk, but with her husband's help she managed to walk downstairs, where she was violently sick. Her husband called for the ambulance, and she was taken to hospital.

She was quickly transferred to a bigger hospital for specialist care. She had a CAT scan, and was prepared for surgery to stem the blood flow in her brain, but the doctors then decided not to operate. She felt dazed for about three days, but was fully conscious. She found she had difficulty eating, because her face was paralysed on the right side. She could speak normally, so she was able to discuss her fears about losing her baby, or dying herself. She remained in hospital for six weeks, and then went home. At that stage, she walked with a Zimmer frame, and her arm was weak, with poor grip, although she could move her fingers normally.

Ike rested at home, and was given daily physiotherapy treatment. Her baby was delivered about a month later at her local hospital under epidural anaesthetic with forceps. He was a healthy boy weighing 6 pounds 9 ounces. Ike's hemiplegia was not worsened by the birth, and she returned home with the baby after the normal period in hospital. Once she was home she resumed physiotherapy treatment, with a physiotherapist visiting her at home. The treatment was aimed at improving Ike's walking, and in particular freeing her from the Zimmer frame. Seven months after her stroke, Ike had a check angiogram, in case she still needed surgery for an aneurysm. A week later, she had an epileptic fit, and was put on tablets. She had three or four fits during the following year, but the fits stopped when the dosage of her anti-convulsant drugs was increased.

Ike managed to bring up her son, despite the difficulties caused by her hemiplegia. The family lived in an isolated farmhouse on hilly ground, so pushing the baby's pram around was a major effort for Ike. Eight months after her stroke, Ike decided to travel to London for specialist physiotherapy treatment and guidance. She attended a specialist treatment centre for a course. Three months later, less than a year after her stroke, she felt fit enough to return to her work as a hairdresser part-time, going in three times a week from 10 a.m. to 4 p.m. She continued to work part-time for over three years, and then returned to full-time working when her son started to go to school.

By this time, she could do virtually everything she used to do before her stroke, including driving, skiing, riding a bicycle, and entertaining. She took her newer role as a mother in her stride, and she and her husband thoroughly enjoyed the child they had waited for for so long. She still felt she could make further progress: she wanted to be able to jump on her bicycle, for instance, without having to think about her balance. She continued to attend for specialist physiotherapy treatment sessions three or four times a year, to ensure that she maintained good control of any residual signs of spasticity.

Ike made an excellent recovery from her stroke, and made the best of it, despite the fact that her circumstances could have been easier. The support she received from her husband helped her motivation to fulfil all the aspects of her life, no matter how difficult. One regret was that she still felt that she wanted another child. She did not think that the pregnancy itself had caused the stroke, and she had been advised that the risk of another stroke was very small, but she was not sure that she could cope with another pregnancy.

Five years after her stroke, Ike remembered the effort of it all as 'bloody hard work', but she advised any young wife, mother or worker to keep trying, and not to 'give in'. Having managed to go skiing, she saw her next challenge as being able to run again, and this was now the ultimate goal of her treatment.

9
Conclusion

We would not pretend that strokes and head injuries are anything other than very serious accidents in a person's life. It would of course be better if they never happened. But as they *do* happen, we would like everyone involved to be aware of the possible after-effects, once the immediate risk of dying is passed. The worst after-effect of brain damage is a hemiplegia which leaves the patient virtually helpless, because spasticity prevents him from using either his damaged side or the normal side effectively. In the best of cases, the patient learns to control the spasticity, and therefore gains the ability to use his body for normal activities. In some cases the recovery is relatively limited, while in others the patient returns virtually to normal. The patient may be able to use the hemiplegic side fully again, or he may be left with a degree of disability, particularly lack of activity in the hemiplegic arm.

Whether the patient remains a helpless prisoner of his spasticity or returns to at least a measure of independence depends entirely on the correct care and handling right from the start of the illness or injury, and accurate, effective rehabilitation during the recovery phases. Motivation is a vital factor: the support and encouragement of a caring family and friends are essential parts of this. The case histories show how much can be done to help the patient regain a useful and enjoyable life, even in the face of severe disabilities. They also show that physical improvement is not limited by time: the patient can go on regaining control and active use of his hemiplegic side for many years after the stroke or head injury. Speech, understanding and perception can also go on recovering over an extended period.

The case histories demonstrate some of the difficulties

patients face. Specialist care and rehabilitation treatment are certainly available in Britain, but proper facilities for this care are very limited. In other European countries, such as Germany and Yugoslavia, patients with brain damage have a statutory right to rehabilitation treatment, and consequently facilities are provided for the purpose. British patients have no such legal rights. There are pitifully few specialist hospitals and rehabilitation centres for brain-damaged patients, and even fewer equipped to modern standards. They can only cater for a small number of patients. If a patient is not lucky enough to receive specialist care through the National Health Service, the only alternative is to pay for private treatment. Therefore, the patient has to be rich enough to pay, or covered by insurance, or prepared to use some of his daily living resources for this purpose. This is hardly a good reflection on the ideal of the British Welfare State.

The lack of specialist facilities is not merely a financial problem. It is also a reflection of some attitudes prevalent within the medical profession. Many doctors still believe that if a stroke or head-injured patient has not made much recovery within a matter of weeks, he will never recover to any reasonable degree. All too often they expect the patient to remain helpless, and to be discharged from hospital to a nursing home for full nursing care and support. They consider rehabilitation treatment a waste of time and money. This attitude totally disregards the scientific work of the neurophysiologists, who have proved beyond doubt that the brain and the nervous system can recover from damage.

Science has backed up the optimism of the rehabilitation specialists, but the knowledge is not yet widely accepted and so put to practical use for all patients. The idea that a brain-damaged person cannot enjoy any kind of worthwhile life, or cannot serve a useful purpose any more is not acceptable in human, social or financial terms. If the patient can be helped to even a small degree of independence, he is less of a burden on his family and the State. While he is trying to improve his condition, he has the in-built reward of seeing his progress. His relationships with other people need not suffer: indeed they may be enriched by the experience of mutual dependence and trust. If the patient returns to normal social and working life, he can continue to make his contribution to society like anyone else. The experience of a stroke or head injury usually serves to show everyone involved how fragile our 'normal' life is, and how quickly and easily it can be disrupted.

We want every patient to be given the chance to make the best of the situation following a stroke or head injury. The hope of recovery is not a vain and idle one if the patient receives the correct support and rehabilitation care from the doctors, nurses, therapists, carers, family and friends. You must never give up hope, even if you have to search for proper care and wait a long time for the results to show. Perseverance and patience will ultimately be rewarded.

Useful Addresses

Banstead Place Mobility Centre
Park Road
Banstead
Surrey SM7 3EE

British Association of Occupational Therapists
6/8 Marshalsea Road
London SE1 1HL

British Sports Association for the Disabled
Mary Glen Haig Suite
34 Osnaburgh Street
London NW1 3ND

BSM Disabled Drivers Training Centre, The
81 Hartfield Road
Wimbledon
London SW19

Chartered Society of Physiotherapy
14 Bedford Row
London WC1R 4ED

Chest, Heart and Stroke Association, The
CHSA House
Whitecross Street
London EC1Y 8JJ

College of Speech Therapists
Herald Poster House
6 Lechmere Road
London NW2 5BU

Department of Health and Social Security
Alexander Fleming House
Elephant and Castle
London SE1 6BY

Disability Information Service Surrey (DISS), The
Harrowlands Park
South Terrace
Dorking
Surrey

Disabled Drivers Association
Registered Office: Ashwellthorpe Hall
Ashwellthorpe
Norwich NR16 1EX

Disabled Living Foundation Equipment Centre
380/384 Harrow Road
London W9 2HU

Garden Club, The
The Gardens for the Disabled Trust
Church Cottage
Headcorn
Kent TN27 9NP

Headway
National Head Injuries Association
17 Clumber Avenue
Sherwood Rise
Nottingham NG5 1AG

'Les Autres Sports'
15 The Binghams
Maidenhead
Berkshire SL6 2ES

Mary Marlborough Lodge
Equipment for Disabled People
Nuffield Orthopaedic Centre
Headington
Oxford OX3 7LD

Medical Branch
Driver and Vehicle Licensing Centre
Swansea SA1 1TU

National Listening Library (Talking Books for the Handicapped)
12 Lant Street
London SE1 1QH

REMAP (Technical Equipment for Disabled People)
25 Mortimer Street
London W1N 8AB

Remploy Ltd
415 Edgware Road
Cricklewood
London NW2 6LR

Royal Horticultural Society, The
80 Vincent Square
London SW1P 2PE

SPOD (Sexual Problems of the Disabled)
286 Camden Road
London N7 0BJ

Index

Index

Index

Index